FRAGILE MINDS

www.penguin.co.uk

Fragile Minds

BELLA JACKSON

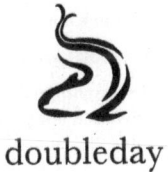

doubleday

TRANSWORLD PUBLISHERS

UK | USA | Canada | Ireland | Australia
India | New Zealand | South Africa

Transworld is part of the Penguin Random House group of companies
whose addresses can be found at global.penguinrandomhouse.com.

Penguin Random House UK, One Embassy Gardens,
8 Viaduct Gardens, London SW11 7BW

penguin.co.uk

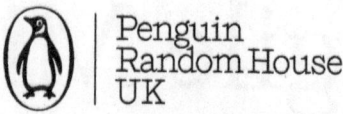

First published in Great Britain in 2025 by Doubleday
an imprint of Transworld Publishers

002

Copyright © Bella Jackson 2025

The moral right of the author has been asserted

Every effort has been made to obtain the necessary permissions with
reference to copyright material, both illustrative and quoted. We apologize
for any omissions in this respect and will be pleased to make the
appropriate acknowledgements in any future edition.

As of the time of initial publication, the URLs displayed in this book link or refer to
existing websites on the Internet. Transworld Publishers is not responsible for, and
should not be deemed to endorse or recommend, any website other than its own or any
content available on the Internet (including without limitation at any website, blog page,
information page) that is not created by Transworld Publishers.

Penguin Random House values and supports copyright. Copyright fuels creativity,
encourages diverse voices, promotes freedom of expression and supports a vibrant culture.
Thank you for purchasing an authorized edition of this book and for respecting intellectual
property laws by not reproducing, scanning or distributing any part of it by any means
without permission. You are supporting authors and enabling Penguin Random House to
continue to publish books for everyone. No part of this book may be used or reproduced
in any manner for the purpose of training artificial intelligence technologies or systems. In
accordance with Article 4(3) of the DSM Directive 2019/790, Penguin Random House
expressly reserves this work from the text and data mining exception.

Typeset in 12/15.5 pt Minion Pro by Jouve (UK), Milton Keynes
Printed and bound in Great Britain by Clays Ltd, Elcograf S.p.A.

The authorized representative in the EEA is Penguin Random House Ireland,
Morrison Chambers, 32 Nassau Street, Dublin D02 YH68.

A CIP catalogue record for this book is available from the British Library

ISBN: 9781529939774

Penguin Random House is committed to a sustainable future
for our business, our readers and our planet. This book is made
from Forest Stewardship Council® certified paper.

For everyone with a story

Contents

Author's Note 1

1. The Door 3
2. The Treatment Room 44
3. The Hallway 77
4. The Bedroom 115
5. The Day Area 147
6. The Beehive 179
7. The Clozapine Clinic 201
8. The Living Room 233
9. The Exit 256

Epilogue 267
Terminology in the UK System 271
Further Reading, Support and Advice 277
Acknowledgements 289

To the thinking mind, which sinks its anchor in the past and future where no anchor will fix, tell this: no things are fixed.

– SAMANTHA HARVEY, *THE SHAPELESS UNEASE*

Author's Note

THIS BOOK HAS BEEN PIECED together from scattered notebooks and scribbles on hands. Scribbles that became long emails to tutors, initially as an attempt to complain, then explain, then just to document.

I have written with the guidance and support of ex-patients, psychiatric survivors and mental health practitioners. The stories I tell here are based on real situations, though the patients, staff and settings are composites and I have gone to some lengths to obscure their identity, changing names, physical details, timelines and histories.

The health care professionals and settings reflect some of the attitudes and approaches of some of the people I encountered during my training. I have given people names to make them come to life but they do not represent or reflect any actual single individual or place of work.

I hope I have done justice to the individuals and their families, and that these stories help amplify the voices of both the rebellious staff and those people who are silenced by their labels – 'disordered', 'dysfunctional' or 'ill'.

I'm aware that I only tell some stories and omit others, that all stories told bear counterbalancing occurrences. I am not refuting those. In the act of recording, I am being biased. I'm showing only a fraction of the whole. But a finished quilt is made from many patches – clashing, partnering, vibrant, faded. Each a unique moment, needing to be acknowledged and remembered.

1

The Door

THE THREE-STOREY BUILDING THAT HOUSED the Acute Psychiatric Ward squatted beside an industrial estate. It looked insignificant from the outside, a blocky, cream-coloured structure with a fresh blue and green sign: Centre for Mental Health Care. As I turned off the pavement towards the sliding entrance doors, a raised bed filled with yellow flowers protruded into view. At its centre, a shrub had been pruned into a lopsided sphere.

It was my first morning on placement as a student mental health nurse. Learning on the job would make up a large portion of my two-year postgraduate training, with university days threaded throughout. The course had started in the classroom three weeks earlier, via introductions and welcome material. To my surprise, I found myself having to articulate to myself as well as to others why I was there.

Why *was* I there? I'd been working in social care for five years and though in many ways this step seemed like a tactical career move, it very much felt like a venture into the unknown. In previous jobs I'd worked regularly with people in mental distress struggling with panic, anxiety, loss. Yet 'mental illness' felt perplexingly delineated from both my life and my work. It existed just out of reach: the clients who were assessed and swiftly directed off elsewhere, the voyeuristic documentary on TV, a garish headline in the newspaper, a man on the bus talking to his reflection in the glass. It seemed perceptible yet frighteningly undefined. Nebulous, it loomed over me; a presence I couldn't shake. What I needed, I reasoned, was to *understand*. To open all the doors into psychiatry and stand right up close to the people within.

The reception area was empty. It looked like any other hospital waiting area: rows of plastic chairs, magazines, innocuous prints of flowers on the walls. I had been expecting something more otherworldly.

A bulky man behind the reception desk was watching me expressionlessly. He nodded.

'Can you sign in?' he asked.

I gave him my details and printed my name on the staff sheet, my heart thudding steadily.

'Wait,' he said, gesturing to my lanyard. 'Is this quick release?'

'Quick what?' I replied.

The man stared at me. 'I'm going to *pull* this,' he said, as if explaining to a child. He clasped the strings around my neck. 'To check it, OK?'

'OK,' I said, unsure.

He gave a short, sharp tug and the lanyard snapped off cleanly. He handed it back to me.

'Good.' He turned to his computer. 'You can go in now.'

His large forearm directed me towards the corridor behind him.

'Right,' I replied, still gripping my lanyard. 'Thank you.'

I followed the corridor, reclipping the loop of fabric around my neck and imagining the consequences of a lanyard that didn't 'release'. Some metres down, I stopped in front of a heavy, air-locked door with a large LCD screen above it. ACUTE WARD scrolled across in luminous, robotic text. Fire engine red. There was a keypad on the right. FOR ENTRY, a button declared in marker pen.

Through the panels of reinforced glass at the centre of The Door, I could see several people milling about in a stretch of hallway. One, a gaunt man wearing a baseball cap, looked at me and frowned enquiringly. Something tangled in my stomach. *I can't hesitate now*, I thought, *I've been seen*. I pressed the button, my heart galloping, as the man began striding towards me.

*

When I was six, I locked myself in the bathroom.

My parents were having a house party, and every room was a jumble of legs. That's how I remember it, as if I'd spent most of the night on the floor or under a table. The voices felt shrill and jarring, the movements of drunken limbs unpredictable and frightening. Someone fell in the pond. The air in our tiny flat was heavy with smoke. I remember crawling around shoes, gripping two of my favourite things in the world: a Sylvanian Families bear and a Kylie Minogue cassette tape.

At some point, I retreated to the bathroom. The stripped wooden door had a chunky iron lock with one of those old-fashioned ornate keys. I turned it smoothly, hearing it click into place, and felt a sense of power, of control. The sound of bass and laughter was dampened there, the unknown adults just shapes moving past the peculiar stained-glass window: I was safe. I had a space which belonged to me, an interlude to verify and identify what I was feeling. Like a pair of lungs expanding, I felt giddy with relief. Locked doors can offer such freedom.

After some time playing in the empty bath with my bear, I stood rejuvenated at the door and clasped the cool iron key. I turned it, and nothing. I tried again, but the door remained locked. Again and again. I can remember the heat flooding my face, my stomach hollowing. In my panic, I didn't think to bang on the door. Didn't want to draw attention to myself, in case I was ignored. That would have been too much to endure. So I stood there for ever, it seemed, turning that key. My hand aching, my ears buzzing with blood. I was crying, shaking. While everyone continued as normal outside. Maybe, I reasoned, they *knew* I was there, had somehow locked the door from the other side. Maybe they wanted me out of the way – it was easier without a child getting under their feet.

When it finally opened, I was despondent with fear and my fantasy of rejection. I was free, but remained abandoned. Just like that, all power had been taken from me, and no one had come to my rescue.

*

The gaunt man was intercepted by a woman with elfin-short hair and glasses, a nurse's lanyard around her neck. She pushed her body between his wiry frame and The Door. I heard her telling him in a muffled voice to step back, then again more sternly. The man took an almost comically large step backwards and grinned.

The woman turned, her teeth catching the light as she smiled.

'You're early!' she pronounced, opening The Door just wide enough for me to slip through. 'I like early people.'

Her accent was soft and lulling, the cadence resting on the first syllable of each word.

I offered the calmest greeting I could manage, while attempting to avoid eye contact with the man peering over her shoulder. She too ignored him and closed The Door behind me. It moved heavily, wading through the warm air before clicking into the frame.

It's easy to walk in and out of a locked ward and forget the significance of that power. Does The Door protect the vulnerable people inside from the unkind world? Or does it protect our fragile society from the people who embody its failings? Perhaps, neither and both are true. What is true, is that having mastery over that portal tugs at many conflicting feelings. Of relief, of self-importance, pride and shame.

'I'm Ray,' the woman said, 'I'm a staff nurse here.'

I followed her down the hallway, the man sloping beside us like a concierge. Slowing, I rebuked myself for ignoring him and caught his eyes hesitantly.

'Hi,' I said, introducing myself.

He echoed me, replacing my name with his own. Hodi.

Ray was talking over him. 'Well, well! Your first placement!' she said. 'This is a good place to start.'

She stopped in front of an office door, the glass obscured from within by a mangled venetian blind. As she sifted through a large bundle of keys clipped to her waist, I took the opportunity to look around me.

Four or five men stood apart from each other, watching us in silence. Looking back, I'm unsure if the ward really did freeze like this, or if it was only my perception of it. As if the only way I could take it in was to isolate everyone like pieces on a chessboard.

My tall acquaintance, Hodi, was the nearest to us. His eyes wide enough to display shock, his willowy eyebrows arching around them. Yet his droll, grinning lips seemed to betray the other features.

Over his left shoulder was a small, heavily stooped man wearing dental-green hospital pyjamas, the bottom half of the ensemble hanging perilously low below his waist. He appeared to be leaning forward on to the balls of his feet, his arms pendulous away from his body, his face a tired waxwork. A flicker of drool hung from the browned front teeth in his open mouth, his eyelids half-mooned and flaccid. I guessed him to be in his late forties, though I later found out he was just thirty-one.

I put up my palm in awkward salutation. The man's eyes followed my hand steadily, but his face remained unchanged. Somewhere within his throat a rush of air curled upwards. Reaching his tongue, it formed a guttural, gurgling reverberation. A slow smile pulled across his face, as if amused by his own incoherence. Then on cue, his trousers slipped down to his protruding knees and hung there. The man continued to sway, his eyes fixed on mine.

The key had been found.

'Come in and put your bag down,' Ray declared, breaking my trance-like state.

'Yes,' I said reflexively, my body following her into the room.

'Jack, pull your trousers up,' she instructed to the closing door.

The other men remained shapes against the blank walls.

*

I have avoided writing about Jack for years; his story still haunts me. My mind often wanders to him, before sharply retreating, like the sudden horror of swimming over an abyss. But I will get to Jack.

*

In the office, Ray explained her role to me. She was mostly kept busy running things behind the scenes, writing up reports for tribunals, organizing admissions and finding staff to cover shifts. But she was still the 'key nurse' for three patients, and said she'd keep an eye on how I was doing.

I handed her my placement booklet and she flicked through the tasks I'd need to complete to qualify. Reading the list at university, I had been surprised by their basic nature. I had to be signed off for such pleasantries as being 'non-judgemental, respectful and courteous at all times when interacting with patients and colleagues' and being 'able to work effectively within the inter-disciplinary team to build professional relationships'. There were more practical tasks to check off too, such as administering medication, taking accurate vital signs, remaining aware of patients' care plans and demonstrating a knowledge of pharmacology. Nurses largely learn their craft from those around them and, as a staff nurse, Ray would play a crucial part in this.

'So . . .' She lingered on the word, watching me. 'You've got a background in social care and counselling?'

I nodded keenly, explaining my various jobs and courses. As we talked, Ray smiled broadly, though her interjections were clipped – as if she hadn't the space in her day for elaborate sentiments – and I felt more scrutinized than reassured.

She closed my booklet and peered at me again. Unsure what she was hoping for, I asked about the number of patients on the ward.

'Twenty-two,' she replied, 'and they're all *very ill*.'

Before I could respond, she clapped her hands together, making me jump.

'Oh yes! We're always at full capacity here.'

She explained that some patients were there 'by choice' – otherwise known as informal admissions – some were detained under Section 2 of the Mental Health Act for twenty-eight days, some on Section 3 for up to six months, while others had been there over a year.

'We'll go through everyone later,' she said, waving the words away. 'You have a wander round and get a feel for the place. Stay within the hallway and day area. Don't go into any bedrooms alone.'

My head was swamped with questions, but I didn't want to look as though I was stalling for time.

'Oh, and there's a psychology group today you should join,' she continued, swivelling slowly from side to side in her chair.

'That would be great!' I enthused, reiterating how interested I was in psychological treatment.

Ray squinted through her glasses at me. 'Look...' she said. 'You're in nursing now. Nursing is about recording and passing on information. Leave the psychology to the psychologists. Your number one role is to keep people safe. If everyone is alive at the end of your day, then you're being a good nurse.'

When I left the office, Hodi, Jack and the rest of the shadow men had gone. Instead, a lone man with a rough beard and greasy hair was pacing towards me. His head curling forward to face the floor, hands knitted together, his feet making no sound on the lino, like a pensive ghoul.

I watched him getting closer, wondering what to say, which way to move, but at the last second he steered around me as a boat avoids a sunken rock. On reaching The Door, he turned fluidly on his heels and started back the other way. This time I managed a 'Hello'.

Several seconds of silence followed as he continued to move away from me. Then, as if my words were a long stick prodding him in the side, the man flinched and looked up with a startled expression.

'Hello?' he asked, his forehead creasing.

And then he was gone, his headless silhouette drifting down the hall.

I decided to get my bearings from somewhere I could stand without looking too conspicuous and headed for the ward's reception area. On my way, I passed a large, glass-fronted room I would come to know as the beehive. Inside, staff members in plain clothes, discernible by their blue lanyards, milled about and chatted. Mental health staff now rarely wear uniforms. This informality is said to aid discreetness when working out in the community, and encourage engagement and trust on wards.

The reception desk was empty, and I hovered behind it, busying myself with reattaching pens to clipboards which had been glued down to the tabletop. On the wall behind the desk I noticed a rack of haphazard, yellowed leaflets and picked one up. *Risperidone – an antipsychotic*, it said. *Do not take this medication with alcohol or 'street' drugs.* I'd never heard of risperidone, and turned the leaflet over in my hand. *It is usually safe to take risperidone*, it continued, *but it's not suitable for everyone. More than one in ten people might get these side effects – headache and movement disorders including tremor, shaking, spasms, problems with speech, unusual movements of tongue, face or other parts of the body that you can't control.* I looked up. *Wait*, I thought – *more* than one in ten? I picked up another leaflet, on benzodiazepines, drugs used mostly for treating anxiety and insomnia. *More than one in ten people might experience side effects of anxiety or agitation, confusion, loss of memory, or dizziness*, I read. Something uncomfortable moved through me.

I shook the feeling off. *OK*, I thought, *I need to be active, I need to go somewhere.*

Around me, bedroom doors were beginning to creak open and drowsy-looking patients were appearing in the hallway, their eyes and lips gummy with sleep. After squaring the leaflets for a fourth time, my heart thudding, I rounded the reception desk and began making my way back to the office to feign some sense of purpose. On my right I passed a large room with the words DAY AREA printed across the open door. Inside, a meandering line of patients was forming for breakfast. A few faces looked up at me blankly.

This is stupid. Just go in. Talk to someone.

I turned and walked into the day area as slowly as I could. A nurse in a crisp white shirt stood just inside the door, a ring of keys secured to his trousers. He smiled at me and nodded, before looking away. I introduced myself, which he seemed to find amusing. 'Yes' was all he said.

I watched the line of patients murmuring and swaying amorphously.

'Hey!' The nurse moved rapidly towards the mass of bodies, his arms flapping. 'Stay in a line!'

A patient in a leg brace glared at him. 'Fuck off,' he said pointedly.

This doesn't seem like the right time to be here, I told myself. *Maybe I'll just go back to the office and read some notes.*

I left the room feeling stiff and pathetic, listening to my new nursing shoes squeaking against the floor. As I turned the corner, The Door and reception desk came back into view. Several patients were now stood around it, their backs to me. One squat, heavy-set man was facing The Door, his body mirrored in the glass panelling, his shaved head glinting under the strip-lights.

A nurse navigated his way around the other patients, before stopping next to him.

'Saul,' I heard him say. 'Saul, can you move away from the door?'

Saul said something I couldn't hear.

'*Saul*,' the nurse said again in a scolding tone. He put his arm on Saul's and tried to guide him backwards.

Saul shook it free. 'I'm fine *here*,' he said loudly.

'Look . . . If you don't want your medication, you'll become *unwell*,' the nurse said. 'Why do you want to see the doctor? You can talk to *me*.'

Saul laughed. 'Hah! Thanks, but no thanks,' he said, still staring at The Door.

Ray appeared, her arms crossed over her chest. 'What's going on?'

The nurse threw up his hands and backed away.

Saul, an East Ender in his late forties, turned to look at her. His face was a deep burgundy, sheened with sweat. There was a tiny, basic mobile phone in his hand.

'I should be *respected*, that's all I ask,' he said.

Ray angled her head. 'OK,' she replied, 'you're being respected. Why are you waiting by The Door?'

'I already *told* him,' Saul said, gesturing to the nurse who was now leaning against the wall a few metres away. 'I want to talk to the doctor about my meds. That's all I fuckin' ask. I WANT to TALK to him.'

Ray smiled. 'Can you talk to me instead?'

Saul started jabbing at the phone with his large hands. 'I'm callin' my lawyer if I can't talk to him. I'm not fuckin' pissin' around.'

'*OK*, Saul,' Ray repeated. 'But you can wait for him *away* from The Door. You'll be called if it's your time for ward round.'

Saul turned and pushed through the other patients, barrelling past me.

The leaning nurse raised his eyebrows and chuckled as he passed.

There was something so unusual, so confusing, about seeing a person in such a heightened emotional state faced with someone so apathetic.

I watched Saul go into his bedroom momentarily, then he came out again.

'Can someone other than *this* guy speak to me?' he pleaded, gesturing with his chin towards the chuckling nurse.

I looked around. Ray had already gone back down the hallway to the office and closed the door. All the other nurses were visible in the beehive, but just out of reach.

'I can – can speak to you,' I said, a little too formally.

I moved towards him, wondering if I was going to be rejected or shouted at as an unknown, a person with clearly no power at all. But Saul nodded, business-like.

'Thank you,' he said.

'Are you . . . OK?' I asked, feeling immediately idiotic.

'Fuckin' . . . no. No,' he said under his breath, 'I'm *not* OK. It's ward round today, but I can't remember if it's my day or not, and no one will fuckin' tell me so I can prepare . . .'

Had I missed something? The request seemed straightforward enough.

'Should I ask for you?'

'Yeah.' He nodded. 'That would be nice.'

I turned from him.

'Hey!' Saul's raised voice echoed off the walls. I spun back round. '*Who are you?*'

'Oh, sorry,' I said. 'I'm just a student nurse.'

'Right. Right.' He began jabbing at his phone again. 'Hello student nurse.'

I asked in the office. It was not Saul's day to meet with the consultant – or 'ward round' as they called it here.

'Well fuckin', fuckin' great. Great!' Saul yelled when I told him. 'It's never my turn is it? I have *things* to say to him. I have things I want to *change* about my medication. No one fuckin' *listens* in here . . .'

A slender, sharply dressed man in a cardigan pushed through The Door and slipped lithely into an office. Dr Oxley, one of the psychiatrists. Saul leapt past me, his phone swinging at his side.

'Doctor!' he yelled. 'When am I seein' you, doctor? I have something to say to you! When am I gettin' *out*?'

He turned to face The Door to the outside world and then to the doctor's office, as if deciding which one to pound on first. He chose the office door. The palm of his hand slapped quickly and incessantly, before winding down to a slow, desperate thump. He paused, waiting.

'Fucker!'

The extreme anxiety around meeting the consultant could be felt by talking with any of the patients. Some spent hours hovering around The Door trying to catch him as he flitted in and out, always with somewhere else to be.

That day there were two other patients waiting for him alongside Saul. One looked glum, the other panic-stricken.

'All right guys,' Saul said, gathering the men conspiratorially.

'I don't think we'll be gettin' anywhere with Fuck Head today, so go get a coffee or somethin'.'

Saul and I talked in the hallway for some time, his eyes darting back and forth between me and the office.

'When people don't speak to you in a *normal* way,' he said, 'don't give you *respect*, it makes you feel sort of inhuman, you know? It's hard to explain . . .'

He tightened his grip on his phone and I worried he would crush it.

'The doctor, all he ever asks me is "How are you feelin' from one to ten?" It's fuckin' ridiculous! He gets paid a lot for doin' that. That and fuckin' druggin' me up with five different meds. Good job I've got a sense of humour.'

A middle-aged man with no front teeth joined our conversation. 'Yeah!' he added, flicking a lock of hair from his face. 'Thing is, prison's better than here. At least with prison you do your time, or less. Then you leave . . . you know when you're getting *out*. Here they can keep you for ever, no idea for how long.'

Saul was nodding. 'That's true! My cousin is out now and he's the most violent man I know. He stabbed two people but they let him out real quick, and now everyone leaves him the fuck alone. No one's stuffin' pills in his face. But *I'm* still locked up, cos I'm *mental* . . . But I never hurt no one. It's not fair.'

After some time, Dr Oxley reappeared, heading at speed towards The Door.

'Doctor!' Saul yelled after him. 'Do you care about people's feelings, doctor? Do you care about anyone?'

Dr Oxley, still propelling forward, looked over his shoulder. 'I hope so!' he exclaimed. And in a second he was gone, The Door closing firmly behind him.

'Bastard!' Saul screamed through the glass.

*

The longest you can be held in a UK prison before being taken to court is fourteen days, which *only* applies to arrests made under the Terrorism Act. Otherwise, a suspected criminal can be held for twenty-four hours, which can be extended to ninety-six hours if the crime is very serious. This is unless you've ever been convicted of a crime in the past, in which case you're likely to be held on remand in prison for up to six months. With suspected mental health conditions, a person can be detained against their will under Section 2 for an initial twenty-eight days for *assessment*. If it's decided you have a mental disorder and you're deemed 'at risk' to either yourself or others and you're not agreeing to the treatment advised, you can be detained for a further six months under Section 3. There is no limit to the number of times Section 3 can be renewed.

When I'd read about the different sections during our introductory weeks, they'd sounded thorough to me, and I'd given them little further thought. But the reality of seeing people confined by these legalities was striking. On a page, the protocols are just cold numbers. In the flesh, the fear and anger that emanates from them is palpable.

*

Later that afternoon, I joined the psychology group Ray had recommended. I was introduced in the hall to Davina, one of the two hospital psychologists. Davina was very thin; her skin looked stretched over her bird-like skull, her glasses balanced on the tip of her nose.

'Come in with me, no problem,' she said, clutching a clipboard to her chest.

There were six of us in the group: Davina, three patients, a trainee psychologist and me. I sat quietly with a pen and paper, and the workshop on Positive Thinking began.

'Today we are going to think about positivity and imagination,' Davina declared. 'We are going to consider how the way people with *healthy* minds get along is that they are able to say "Yes" to challenges and opportunities that arise, rather than people with *disturbed* minds who cannot do this . . .'

My body became rigid. I looked around the circle. *Disturbed minds?* The trainee psychologist sat placidly, her eyes fixed on Davina.

'Now,' Davina continued, 'shall we introduce ourselves?'

Her eyes rested on a fidgety, rotund man staring at the floor. Vern presented himself dutifully, telling us his name and diagnosis: paranoid schizophrenia. He nodded rhythmically as he spoke, his expression empty. Beside him was the pacing man I'd seen when I first came in.

'Schizoaffective disorder' was all he said.

There was a pause.

'And your name?' said Davina.

There was another pause. The man stared at her in silence.

'OK, *fine*.' Davina shook her hair as if an insect had landed there. 'And who's next?'

Saul sat slumped in his chair, his eyes struggling to stay open.

'Saul,' he told her. 'And I can't fuckin' think straight, just feelin' drugged up.'

'OK, so!' Davina began.

'I've got *too many* diagnoses to say,' Saul continued. 'No fuckin' idea what any of it means.'

The trainee psychologist was smiling and nodding. Saul closed his eyes and broke into a phlegmy snore.

Davina rotated towards Vern again. He appeared to shrink under her gaze.

'And what do you think about what I said, Vern?'

'What?' he said, his eyes widening.

'Of being able to say "Yes" to things, Vern?'

Everybody turned to him.

Silence.

Vern was staring at the floor. 'Yes, that sounds right,' he murmured.

Davina continued, almost triumphantly now. 'Can you see that you were able to say "Yes" to something today, to coming to this group?'

'I guess so,' Vern replied flatly.

Davina leant forward in her chair. '*Today* we are going to use the power of our *imaginations* to take us to a happy, safe place. To focus only on the positive in times of difficulty. Finding a happy place can be like a medicine to combat depressive feelings . . .'

Saul shifted in his armchair, one eye opening. There was a thin line of spittle on his chin.

'Shall I tell you what *I* think?' he began, his voice slurred. 'I think we aren't bein' helped. I think we're bein' *sedated*. Drug companies are makin' a lot of money from our hell.'

Saul's eyes searched the other faces in the room, seeking support, but getting none.

After a pregnant pause, Davina smiled. '*OK*, but this afternoon, Saul, we are focusing on *positive* things not negative things. Isn't that right, Vern?'

Vern looked startled and uttered his response to his shoes: 'That's right . . .'

I must have disengaged at this point. My only memory is of a bodily sensation, one of being pressed hard against the chair by some asphyxiating force. I remember that Saul refused to go to a happy place. That Saul continued his tirade. That Saul was told to be quiet, or to leave. That Saul left us.

The rest of the day passed with brief greetings and a hurried lunch break. Late afternoon, I was invited to Vern's ward round meeting. I joined Dr Oxley, a pharmacist and two staff nurses around a large table in the office. These meetings, I was told, were meant to occur for each patient every two weeks, with the aim of evaluating treatment, progress and discussing care plans from the perspective of both staff and patient. I'd soon learn that in reality patients were lucky if they took place once a month.

I was the last in the room, and a staff nurse introduced me to the rest of the team. Everyone smiled. Up close, Dr Oxley looked almost boyish, his clothes immaculately tucked and pressed. He greeted me politely but remained stony-faced.

As I was finding a seat, there was a tentative knock on the door. I gestured towards it, and, getting a nod of authorization, stood up and opened it.

Vern stepped in, his expansive shoulders filling the doorway. He glanced around the table, sweating profusely, looking even more nervous than he had done in the psychology group. He regarded me without recognition and smiled, offering me his hand.

'Hello, doctor,' he said. His hand was clammy.

I corrected him and pointed towards Dr Oxley, whose facial expression remained unchanged.

'Sit down,' the doctor said.

The other staff were silent. Vern pulled a chair out, and it jolted in his hands.

Dr Oxley looked down at his papers and shuffled through them. He then proceeded to outline how long Vern had been on the ward and checked through his drug chart with the pharmacist. It seemed like an eternity before he looked up for the first time at the man in front of him.

'So,' he began, 'why do you think you were brought here, Vern?'

Vern folded and refolded an invisible piece of paper in his shaking hands. He talked in fragments about his father beating him, his homelessness, his anxiety with others, his loneliness and recurring nightmares. Dr Oxley went back to shuffling papers and glancing over charts as if Vern was absent, his answer left unacknowledged. I felt myself staring openly at the doctor, my mouth so dry that I was struggling to swallow. As Vern's account slowed, the doctor finally looked up again.

'And what *is* the illness that you have?' he asked.

Vern's face crumpled. I could feel my lungs taking in air sharply.

'Erm, erm . . .' Vern was looking at his knees now. His shoulders slumped forward. 'Paranoid schizophrenia, doctor.'

The nurse next to me seemed to rouse from her stupor and on the blank page in front of her she wrote the words 'Vern – paranoid schizoid'.

Vern, who was sitting next to her, saw the note. His face fell.

'Right, paranoid schizophrenia,' the doctor was saying. 'And why do you take your medication, Vern?'

'Because . . .' Vern squirmed in his chair. 'Because of my moods, to make me get better.' He looked up, his eyes rimmed with red. 'But the thing is, sometimes it makes my whole body feel tight, and in my chest . . . a pain . . . I don't feel . . .'

Dr Oxley interrupted him. 'Why did you stop taking your medication at home, Vern? Why do you need to keep taking it?'

'Because – it's making me get better, doctor,' Vern repeated.

'And, do you think you should be discharged?'

Vern's eyes widened. 'Erm, I don't know. I think so. Although, I mean, I'm relying on you doctors and nurses to kindly tell me when I'm well. I'm doing everything I should do.' Vern looked at the pile of paper in front of the doctor. 'I mean, does me not feeling well need to be monitored? My chest? My heart . . . My . . .'

Dr Oxley took a deep breath. 'Well, this is the first time I'm meeting you, but your nurse tells me you've agreed to take the paliperidone injection now instead of the 4mg of risperidone, correct? Which I think will be good for you.'

Vern was nodding. 'Yes. Yes. OK. That sounds OK . . . and then maybe I can leave? If I do that?'

I noticed his knuckles were pale from gripping the table, his large body shifting from side to side in his chair.

'We'll see,' the doctor said.

Vern's body was visibly twitching now, as if the chair had grown hot under his skin.

'Thank you, thank you,' he muttered, standing up, then sitting down abruptly. 'Can I leave now, doctor?'

Dr Oxley handed the file back to the pharmacist. 'You can leave,' he said to the table.

Everyone muttered a goodbye in Vern's direction.

The door closed.

I turned my head back to find Dr Oxley staring at me. His eyes a pale almond colour. The others sat motionless. Everyone silent, waiting. I felt my stomach plunge.

'Just a word of *advice*,' he began, his voice low. 'Do *not* shake these guys' hands. Do *not* smile so much. These men are *psychotic*. Many of them are sexually disinhibited. You don't know how they will take it – or what they will think of you.'

He turned back to his pile of papers, and there was silence again. My heart thudding.

'Come in,' he called to the door, his face down. 'Will someone get that, please?'

An hour later I was first out of the room, mumbling a thank-you-for-having-me to the team. I swallowed hard, pushing through the hallway, my head down. My eyes were stinging as I reached The Door and pressed my staff pass to the exit pad.

In the outside reception, I headed straight to the toilet and found a cubicle, locking it behind me. Suddenly faint, I sat on the lid and cradled my head in my hands. And then, like a hefty club finding its mark, a dull sadness defeated me and I started to sob.

After collecting myself, I let myself back on to the ward. The hallway was quiet, and I made my way to the office. I could feel my heart hammering in my throat as I knocked on the door, not knowing who else to speak to.

'One minute please.' Ray's voice.

I waited, shifting my weight from foot to foot, like a boxer preparing for the ring. The blind swung to one side and Ray's face appeared behind the glass. She smiled.

As soon as I stepped into the room, I felt my eyes start to well again. I told Ray about Dr Oxley, about how he was with Vern, how it all *just didn't feel right*. Ray was nodding, her mouth pulled into an odd shape. The gesture confused me, and I stuttered into silence.

'He shouldn't have said that.' Her face was still unreadable. 'Not in that way at least . . .'

I nodded, relieved. 'Something is wrong . . . with how he is, with how he behaves.' I felt my breathing quicken.

Ray leant forward. 'You must try and disconnect the man himself from the man as a professional,' she said. 'He said that because he means well, he's not a *bad* man. He's just wanting you to be cautious, to be safe here. It's his job, ultimately, to make sure nothing happens to you. That's a lot of pressure.'

This was not what I wanted to hear. I didn't want to reason with him. I didn't want to understand. I realized then that I wasn't just upset about what he had said to me, I was upset about everything I was seeing.

'You know,' Ray continued, 'when Vern was at home, he

stopped taking his medication and smashed his mum's house up. That's why he's here.'

I let this sink in.

'Why?' I asked. 'Because of his chest—'

Ray frowned. 'What do you mean? He stopped taking his medication because he's *mentally ill.*'

I thought of Vern, his fearful child-like face, his trembling hands.

Ray had stopped smiling. 'And Saul,' she continued, 'he beat his girlfriend up before coming in here. They were beating each other up, *actually*. Look . . .' She took a breath. 'Vern, and all these patients, can be very dangerous, don't forget that.'

I nodded slowly, incredulous. Something indescribable had shifted in me that afternoon. A switch had flicked, though to what I didn't know yet.

Leaving the hospital when my shift ended was like tumbling out into a different dimension. Everything felt pale and insignificant in comparison to the lurid, racing movie reel of that ward. Time outside had a different quality: sluggish, flimsy. I remember nothing of the intricacies of how I got from the train to the shower to my bed. Who I saw, what we said to each other.

Several days passed on the ward, a disquiet rising like bile at the back of my throat, before I was back at university for a morning of lectures. I walked into that prestigious building with an uneasy discomfort turning my stomach. Something in me had altered. As students described their placements as 'interesting' and 'exciting' I stared at them, baffled, studying their moving features like a Martian. *Am I doing this all wrong?* I thought. *Is there something wrong with me?*

After class, I sat in the corridor sipping lukewarm tea from the vending machine. Crowds of students moved past me, their bodies blurring together, their voices shrill. I could feel my limbs trembling, my breathing short. I'd been replaying the conversations with my classmates over and over in my head. *I'm angry*, I realized. *I'm really fucking angry.*

A short man with a full yellow beard was weaving his way through the throng. I watched his T-shirt – emblazoned with the image of a demonic-looking, red-eyed Theresa May – moving towards me. Smiling, he sat down and introduced himself as Alex.

We talked for some time about our placements. Alex, like others in our group, had been a health care assistant before enrolling on the course and he now seemed torn between the two roles; speaking of nurses as if they were other to him, his camaraderie still with the assistants he saw as shouldering the bulk of the work. There was a vigorous exuberance to his attitude, an almost giddy joy in the shocking things he'd witnessed on wards; a sense that what he was seeing was proof that life was inadequate and unfair. This confirmation induced a profound relief within him: there was something tangible to fight. Alex had conceived of a purpose and settled on a warming, driving anger to replace the desolation.

'But that's just it,' he was saying. 'Our mental health is always going to be shitty under capitalism. Ideally, you uproot the whole system, bring down those in power – then everything can transform.'

I looked at him, his cheeks pink with enthusiasm.

I would come to relish Alex's sweeping statements about capitalism and corruption being the problem with our psychiatric system, which made most people around him groan. He would laugh off their ridicule, pointing out examples from history or quoting a theory I hadn't heard. I liked him immediately, and felt relieved to find a companion via our mutual interrogative stance. I remained intrigued, however, by what appeared to be his passivity in the face of an experience that deeply distressed me. Instead, these experiences seemed to strengthen and invigorate Alex, to confirm his belief in the system's brokenness and our potential to make the world better. Sometimes his indiscretion made me wince, but he didn't give a fuck. It was refreshing.

'Anger is a *good thing*,' he told me. 'We *need* to be angry about this.'

'I don't know,' I replied. 'Maybe I'm being too idealistic?'

'No, no.' He shook his head. 'Anger will drive the revolution. Seriously. We need anger to make things change.'

We sat and spoke for a while, and I watched as the initial burst of vitriol disappeared, leaving him smiling and flushed again. I envied his ability to shake off experiences, to refuel and spark again and again. Could I do the same?

The next day, feeling less isolated, I returned to the ward and met William by The Door. A returner, I was told he'd been under Section 3 now for almost a month. There was a familiarity to his relationship with the space around him. At least a foot taller than everyone else, his formidable frame seemed constrained within the warren-like hallways, reminding me of Alice after drinking from the mysterious bottle and filling the White Rabbit's home with her swelling limbs.

I watched him throughout the morning, avoiding other patients and staff by turning smartly on his heels when they approached. His long, sloping gait had enough speed to seem purposeful, as though he desperately longed for somewhere to be.

On the few occasions when I was able to speak to him he appeared ambushed and bereft of his solitude, his mournful face examining my own just long enough for me to question whether I'd said something unintelligible. Then he'd answer with a string of mysterious statements, raise a single eyebrow and skulk off again.

Just before lunch, William strode over to the reception desk where I was standing. I caught my breath, hoping this was my opportunity to learn more about him. I watched his long features glide past me and hover over the Patient Leave clipboard, where he peered at the page as though studying his own reflection. Without looking up, he gripped a pen and spelt out I WANT RELEASE in misshapen capitals. Then he lifted the topmost sheet of paper and printed the same words on the next page. And then the next, and the next.

I asked him if he was OK. William's face remained at a right angle to my own.

'I want out,' he replied. 'OUT.'

I looked at the pen shaking in his hand.

'But,' he continued, 'I can't make a fuss or . . . they'll *inject me*.' He looked steadily over his shoulder, then back at the clipboard. 'This place is jinxed. Jinxed!' he said to the pen in his fist. 'I have to get out.' He lifted his head abruptly, his eyes meeting mine for the first time. '*You* have to get out!'

I felt myself blinking, unsure how to answer him as he leant in closer, conspiratorially.

'I want you to call me *Simon Simon* from now on.'

I paused. 'Why?'

William's eyes widened. 'Why not?'

I looked at him. He nodded and slunk away.

William, I found out, had been refusing his medication. Each day he would accept his mood stabilizer, while taking the antidepressant out of the paper pot and placing it carefully on the sideboard.

'No thank you, I'm fine,' he would say. 'I don't need that, I'm perfectly happy.'

The nurse on medication round would spend some twenty minutes attempting to get him to take it, to no avail.

Once a week, William's aunt came to visit. That afternoon she arrived at The Door smiling. He greeted her in the hallway, coming to a halt some feet away, a large grin pulled across his face, one palm in the air in salute.

'William!' she called.

I watched a senior nurse walking towards them. As she passed William, she put her hand gently on his arm. He flinched.

The nurse explained to William's aunt that William *would not* be allowed out that day as he had *not been agreeing* to take his medication. His aunt was nodding, her face a mass of concerned creases. She looked from the nurse to William and back again, saying, 'Oh . . . Oh . . . Oh,' her fingers kneading her shoulder bag.

The nurse turned to William and, lowering her voice as if

speaking to a toddler, said, 'It's just a little tablet . . . just take it quickly all in one go and then you can see your aunt. Do you *understand* me?'

William looked fixedly at her. I could see his chest rising and falling beneath his T-shirt.

'Yes, I *understand* you,' he said. 'I just don't *agree* with you.'

When the nurse left, William and his aunt stood talking in the hall. She continued to nod to herself as she spoke, her gloved hand wiping tears from her cheeks. William's face remained still, his eyes unmoving. Then, without warning, he turned his back to her, his pace now more of a saunter as he edged away down the hallway. As he passed the nurse he did an elaborate bow, his long arm stretching out to one side.

William's aunt made her way towards me, her eyes swollen, her mascara smeared in vertical stripes like badly executed theatre make-up. She told me she was unsure what to do, that she wondered whether William might be autistic as he'd been this way since childhood. She told me she'd asked many times that he be assessed for autism, but that psychiatrist after psychiatrist had told her that for William, in his early fifties, it was 'too late' for an assessment, that there was 'no point'.

I felt an anger rising up through my body and looked at my feet, then at her. 'I'm so sorry,' I heard myself say. 'I'll ask someone about that. I'll . . . ask someone. That's not – that shouldn't be the case.'

William's aunt smiled weakly and wished me a good day. She pressed the tiny letters of her name on to the mangled page of the visitors' book and waited for the buzzer to release her into the world. I watched her walking away, her chin on her chest, her left hand covering her eyes like a hood.

*

An increasing number of studies highlight the prevalence of people on the autistic spectrum being misdiagnosed with a variety of mental health conditions, the most common being mood disorders, psychosis and personality disorders. A continuing lack of autism knowledge and awareness by mental health professionals perpetuates the problem, with women and non-binary people even more likely to be misdiagnosed. Misdiagnosis is shown to be extremely damaging, with people encouraged or forced to take unnecessary medication and to see themselves as ill and in need of medical intervention. This can leave them stuck in an unending cycle of medication and sectioning, without progress.

*

Why wasn't William being given access to an autism assessment if his family requested it? How did he come to be locked in here without all other avenues being explored? I was baffled, and again sought out Ray in the office. She shook her head as if I were making a joke.

'Oh, families will *often* say things like that,' she said. 'They don't want the stigma of the actual illness.' She paused. 'Don't worry, someone before you will have made an informed decision.'

*

The hours passed, and through the window at the back of the beehive I could see the world had fallen into darkness. I stood in the empty strip-lit hallway, watching the clock, my shift almost over. The evening medication had dragged most patients to bed or slumped them on sofas, and a latent hush had descended. Ray put her hand on my shoulder. I jumped.

'Oh!' she said. 'Sorry to stress you! I thought you saw me coming.' She smiled. 'I want you to meet someone.'

We walked together down the hallway, my shoes squeaking into the quiet.

'She's an *interesting* case, Irene,' Ray whispered to me. 'Delusional disorder. Very difficult to treat.'

I hadn't come across the diagnosis before. It sounded vague.

'What are the delusions she has?' I asked.

Ray leant towards me. 'Oh, lots of different delusions.' She looked undecided, her eyes creasing at the corners in thought. 'Delusions around water, around food being poisoned, about evil spirits and things like that. Her son was concerned about her paranoid behaviour at home and contacted the police. They ended up bringing her in. *Boy* did she resist.'

As we rounded the corner, I saw a woman sat alone in the hallway on a dining chair. Her face was angled away from us, looking towards the fire door that led to the courtyard beyond. Her grey hair was piled on top of her head, neatly pinned with silver clasps that twinkled in the strip-lights. I noticed her hands smoothing the creases of her red dress. It had been decades since psychiatric patients were forced to wear hospital gowns. They, like staff, were permitted to wear their own clothes to foster a sense of dignity and personhood.

We stopped and stood together, watching her in silence.

'She's from *Cameroon*,' Ray whispered. I nodded, and Ray began to back away down the corridor. 'I'll let you get to know her a little, then we can discuss your thoughts after.'

I could feel myself frowning, unsure what she was tasking me with. Ray turned, and I watched her hair bouncing in rhythm with her footsteps.

When I looked back, Irene was glaring at me.

'Yes?' she said, as if I were a cold caller at her door. 'How can I *help* you?'

I introduced myself and explained that I was a student.

'Oh?' she asked brightly, turning her small frame towards me. 'And what are you studying?'

'Um,' I faltered, uncomfortable. 'Mental health nursing.'

There was a pause.

'That's interesting.' She squinted at me. 'Mental illness is *complicated*. And what do you want to *do* with yourself when you finish?'

I felt as though I was speaking to my own grandmother, checking in on me, making sure I was planning for the future. Her milky eyes were staring into mine.

'I guess I'm not exactly sure yet . . .' I fumbled, looking back at her.

She angled her head to one side. 'And . . . what *is* mentally ill?' she asked slowly. 'What is actually wrong?'

My thoughts churned, grasping at fragments.

'Well . . .' I began hesitantly. 'It will be . . . really be a . . .'

Irene had clasped her hands together. Her body started to rock. I stared, transfixed.

'*You*,' she said, her finger pointing stiffly, 'you *have* to look *deeper.*' Her lips were puckered. 'It's not as though, ooooh, this old lady can't keep her house in *order*. So? What does she need?' She was almost spitting the words now. '*Support*. That's what she needs! Not to be called *mentally ill*.'

I thought she was going to stand up and begin marching up and down the hall, but she stayed seated, unmoving.

'Look . . .' she continued. 'I've been living here for almost forty years. My husband died four years ago, leaving me alone. *Alone*. In that big old house. No one came. No one helped. They just wanted me gone.' She pursed her lips again. '*Mmm, hmm*. And I *love* this country. They gave me an education when I'd never had one. I went back to my country and felt proud that I'd learnt all these new things. Now . . . now . . .' Her index finger was pointing at me again. 'Let me tell you, I'm not so sure about this country any more.'

There was a pause, and Irene seemed to start breathing again. Her gaze fell away from me and rested on the floor. She shook her head wistfully.

'You know,' she said, her voice softer now, 'I should never have told those people about the evil spirit.'

I felt my head move. She noticed and smiled wryly.

'Oh *yes* . . .' she said. 'The African lady and her evil spirits, yes? What a story for all you white folk.'

I shifted my feet, suddenly aware of my limbs, unsure what to say. Ashamed to acknowledge the stereotype in my mind.

'Oh yes,' she said again. 'He was a boy who robbed me. How he got into my house, I don't know. But he kept coming in and taking things, I'm sure of it.' She studied my face. 'Back in my country, we have spirits. You know this, I think.'

I nodded.

'But!' she continued. 'My son put me here, and my daughter. They want my house, you see. They're angry with me because I left everything to my grandson in my will and not to them. I didn't want to give it to them because they're both *trouble*. They have big problems, money problems. My son – I can't even start. But, sure, I wasn't coping with my housework, things got too much, and they came round and told me I am mad. *Mad*. They called the police on me, had me pulled out of my own home, in front of all the neighbours...'

I shook my head; it sounded distressing. Then I remembered her diagnosis: *delusional disorder*. Something in me stirred. Could I trust anything Irene was saying? Without prior knowledge of the diagnosis attached to her, it all seemed so understandable, so plausible.

'Are you... worried about the water and the food?' I asked.

Irene pretended to spit on the floor. 'Bah! I don't drink tap water – it's full of chemicals, it's poison. And the food! The food here... they're trying to poison me with this filth.'

She knitted her fingers together in her lap.

'Bah,' she said again. 'All that stuff from the microwave is dangerous. This is a prison. They won't even let me go shopping!'

I found Ray in her usual spot in the office. She turned on her chair and peered at me over her glasses.

'Well?' she asked.

I heard myself swallowing. 'She seems kind of, kind of well to me.'

Ray squinted. '*Oh*,' she said carefully. 'She's a smart woman, for sure. But you have to be clever too when assessing someone, you can't let yourself be sucked in.'

I paused, unsure how to respond to this. Was she asking me *not* to make my own assessment? Insinuating that to see Irene as anything other than delusional was *my* error? Believing that she was well felt as plausible as insinuating that she was cleverly deceptive, so how could any kind of recovery be deciphered?

'But,' I said, 'her delusions seemed to be . . . kind of reasonable. At least, they didn't really seem like delusions.'

Ray folded her arms and looked at me, tilting her head in her characteristic way. 'Remember, a professional before you has done a more detailed assessment, and you can't ignore that. They've given you a map to use, so use it.'

I left the office feeling like the wind had been knocked out of me. What kind of agency could nurses have here? Surely with something so subjective – phenomenologically and culturally – as being considered *mentally sane*, staff would be encouraged to query, to investigate? Or was it our job to just toe the line?

A few days later, Irene was granted a trip to the bank accompanied by a health care assistant.

When I returned from lunch there was a flurry of activity outside the beehive, with patients and staff jostling to peer in through the glass. Behind it, a short bald man wearing a smart-looking jacket was talking animatedly to a cheery-looking woman wearing a Hawaiian print dress, her hands conjuring something in the air around her. The man, too, was smiling, but his hands were making slicing motions. Then I noticed Irene behind him, her stance solid, looking more powerful than I'd ever seen her.

A slight, open-faced nurse in a yellow shirt turned to me. 'I'm Fuad,' he said, smiling and offering me his hand. 'Look at this,' he continued, nodding in Irene's direction. 'They were considering a depot, can you believe.'

Depot. I knew the word from my introductory weeks. An injection containing antipsychotic medication deposited in the muscle tissue that slowly seeped into the body over a number of weeks. It was often used to enforce 'compliance' when there was concern over whether a patient would agree to take medication orally.

'Wow,' I said, noting his scepticism with a pulse of relief. It seemed like a drastic decision for someone as passive as Irene.

'Yeah,' Fuad continued. 'She hasn't touched any medication since she's been here, and they weren't sure what to do. Luckily, Dr McCulloch's her consultant.'

I looked at him. 'Dr McCulloch?'

He nodded. 'That's her there in the dress. She actually takes the time to consider, which is more than I can say for, well . . .' He paused, frowning. 'But, sadly,' he added, shaking his head, 'she's here, there and everywhere. She's locum.'

I watched the bald man push his sleeves up his arms.

'So, what's going on?' I asked.

Fuad turned to me, his eyebrows raised. 'Oh, you didn't *hear*?' he answered, his voice rising. 'On the way to the bank, Irene bolted off the bus and into the Cameroonian Embassy. Started screaming that she'd been kidnapped and held hostage. Refused to leave without the ambassador accompanying her to ask for discharge.'

I turned to him. '*No.*'

He grinned. 'Oh *yes*. That's him in there with them.'

I watched Irene, her elbows jutting out from her hips in a combative stance.

'Irene's lucky Dr McCulloch's here,' Fuad whispered. 'Stuff would have hit the fan if she wasn't.'

I watched the doctor smiling, her hand now on the ambassador's shoulder. They both laughed at something.

'Is this pretty unusual?' I asked. 'I mean, Irene's on a Section Two, right? She's not an informal patient?'

Fuad's eyes remained fixed on the mime behind the glass. 'Yeah,' he said. 'But embassies are foreign soil, I think. Pretty crafty of her.'

We stood silently, transfixed. A nurse pressed her way through the bodies and past us, huffing under her breath. She stopped and followed our gaze. Taking in the scene, she tutted loudly and moved on.

Beyond the glass, the meeting was ending. The three now appeared to be dancing round each other, shaking hands. Irene was beaming. I turned to Fuad and he too was smiling broadly.

'*Huh*,' he said, shaking his head. '*Well*.'

The door to the beehive swung open and Irene and the ambassador walked out together, their elbows clearing a path through the crowd. There was a small leather suitcase in Irene's hand, her face resolute. As she moved past us, a patient jolted towards her.

'Get me out!' he yelled, before being pulled briskly back by a nurse.

Irene turned to him. 'I'm sorry, boy,' she said.

The ambassador and Irene stopped together at The Door,

waited until a buzzer sounded, and stepped into the outside world. The Door closed heavily behind them.

I watched them disappear around the bend.

'Good for her,' Fuad said. 'I never trusted that son of hers anyway. It was probably a load of bull all along.' He looked at me. 'See you about,' he said, smiling. 'I'm in most days.'

With the entertainment over, staff and patients dispersed. I stood still, aware of the space opening around me, and felt flooded with white light.

How was it possible that things had changed in a heartbeat for Irene? How was it so easy for the decision about release to go either way – depending on the consultant, the opportune moment?

The tutting nurse moved off to the reception desk where she sat down heavily, her forearms propped on the surface.

'Well,' she said loudly to no one in particular, 'I guess no depot for *her* then.' She peered up at me, taking me in. 'Can you check some patient vitals now, please,' she said, using my name, despite my never having spoken to her. 'And then you can help reorganize the fridge. It's not all about *one-to-ones* here, you know.'

Her face was pinched and sour. I watched her flip open a laptop and begin scouring a Wikipedia page on medication side effects.

'Or,' she added, her back to me, 'I can find something else for you to do.'

At the end of my first two weeks on the ward I wrote an email to one of my tutors, Clement. I had been taking notes continually since I'd arrived, scribbling down my incomprehension and shock. Compiling what I had seen felt like the only way to convey what was happening. I needed to be less alone with it, but much more than that, I needed validation: to know if my confusion and anger were justified. After all, I argued with myself, I was an outsider. Perhaps my incredulity was mistaken?

After reading my email, Clement rang me at home.

'*Ah.*'

Clement had a way of saying everything while saying nothing at all. Since leaving mental health nursing almost ten years earlier, he had moulded himself unequivocally into an academic, and he now made it his mission, it seemed, to talk to people as little as possible.

'Ah?' I echoed, wanting something solid from him.

'Definitely less than ideal,' he offered.

I wanted comfort, suddenly. I wanted him to direct me, tell me exactly what to do. 'I feel like I can't . . . I don't know if I can . . .'

Like a bloodhound sensing a whiff of heightened emotion, Clement steered the conversation ninety degrees. 'It's honestly not worth trying to complain at this point,' he said. 'Difficult to illustrate that I'm not being yellow-bellied here, but it will cause you a huge amount of hassle and fight which you won't win. I've seen it many times.'

I took this in. 'Are you sure?'

'Well,' he said haltingly. 'What you're describing is definitely bad practice . . . It's very interesting actually.'

His voice sounded buoyant somehow.

'Though the thing is, when I say *bad practice*,' Clement continued, 'it's not actually bad *enough* for anyone to take it any further. Everyone will deny everything, back each other up, and nothing is sufficiently concrete anyway. It would probably make things more difficult if you reported it.'

'Oh...'

'You see,' he went on, 'everyone seems to know everyone in the mental health world. And really, it's hard to get people fired, even if they really ought to be. They just move them to another ward. I saw it happen all the time, even to staff who were doing much, much worse than you described.'

'Really? But – why weren't they fired?'

Clement described a myriad of vague systemic problems, from staff shortages to Kafkaesque policies. He lamented private health care operatives who he warned were even worse than the NHS, often taking on staff the NHS had disciplined for malpractice. I felt stunned. It could almost be farcical if it wasn't so horribly, deeply upsetting.

'It's generally a bad situation all round,' he summarized. 'And especially hard for the poor patients to complain – they're not usually coherent enough to make a good case.'

I looked out of the window to the street beyond. A shaft of sun was breaking through the clouds; someone cycled past with a bunch of flowers in their front basket. Relief washed over me, followed by a grip of shame. I could leave the ward, go back to my home, make decisions about what I would and wouldn't do with my day, with my life.

'I just, I don't know what to do. It all feels really wrong, and I don't know if I can—'

'I *think*,' Clement interrupted, 'there is something important about writing it all down.' His voice sounded animated again. 'I think the best thing you can do now is continue recording what you witness, and then we'll see what we've got. I think maybe we'll treat this like *research*, and then we'll have another think.'

I put the phone down, feeling drained. My concern about the treatment I was witnessing wasn't yet coherent and I'd wanted Clement to instruct me through something procedural. But maybe he was right, maybe nothing could be done at this point. Or, maybe, I reasoned, I misunderstood something fundamental, lacked some kind of knowledge that would make everything clear? Perhaps there would be a moment, somewhere within the course, when I'd learn enough to slot in like a coin, all discomfort leaving me? When I'd go about my day as the other staff seemed to? After all, I was only a student nurse. Surely everything would make sense with more time?

I spent that weekend at home, writing. My body hunched at the dining room table, my mind disoriented, still sealed within the ward. While asleep, I'd re-enact arguments with Dr Oxley. I'd give long, perfectly articulated reasons for my dislike of him, as the walls began to writhe beneath the paint. In the depths of my dream, the lino floor would shift and darken beneath my feet, a revulsion pulsing through my body as the panic took hold, like the claws of some enormous beast. And suddenly I was immobile, as inconspicuous as a light fitting, as dull-eyed people dragged themselves from room to room like corpses, as pills were dispensed, injections prepared, doors locked.

2

The Treatment Room

IT WAS WEEK FOUR, AND morning handover was about to begin in the beehive. I watched quietly as staff filtered in and rotated impatiently on office chairs or typed vigorously at computers. This ritual had started to feel routine, the patterns and habits revealed through familiarity.

'*Who's* coming?' one nurse asked, leaning across to another.

'You know him,' the other nurse replied. 'With the *hats*.'

The first nurse looked puzzled, then amused. 'Oh, yeah.'

'He's a peer support worker, you know?' the other nurse said, nodding. 'He's got a blog and everything.'

'*Is he?*' The first nurse laughed. 'Oh, we'd better be a bit careful then.'

Ray stopped typing and made a mock-scolding face at the two nurses. 'We'll treat him *exactly* as we treat everyone else,' she said, before turning to me. 'You didn't hear that.' She winked.

Outside the glass I could see Hodi, the sloping concierge from my first day on the ward, pacing back and forth, calling Ray's name. Again and again.

'Welcome and hi.' Ray stood up, her back to Hodi, raising her hands like a conductor. 'Let's begin,' she called out to the room. 'Shall we?'

As the meeting progressed with descriptions of patients, changes in sectioning and allocation of daily tasks, I watched Hodi's gangly body lumbering up and down the hallway outside, always on the move, his capped head popping in and out of view.

Over the previous weeks I'd noticed his primary mode of engagement was to ask questions: *Why did they hang that sign there? Why does he always use a red pen? Can you tie shoelaces better than me? Can you explain this word to me? Why do you flick your hair?* Many of the staff seemed irritated by him. They called him 'attention-seeking' and 'intrusive', two adjectives that came up regularly in his notes, which I'd spent some time reading. His diagnosis appeared scrambled: personality disorder, schizoaffective disorder, unspecified-mood-disorder-with-psychotic-tendencies. He was prescribed two antipsychotics, plus one benzodiazepine and a sedative-hypnotic. The only drug action outlined clearly was the sedative-hypnotic, which was for sleep. The antipsychotics were unexplained in his notes, as was the lorazepam, which I knew to be mostly used for anxiety, or as a sedative. In psychiatry, the same drugs are prescribed for a multitude of different symptoms and it can be challenging to tease apart which drug is meant to treat what. This lack of clarity for both patients and staff was frustrating. How had this decision been made? How was it that the consultants so readily disagreed on diagnosis or prescription?

The end of handover rolled around.

'Raaay!' Hodi was still pacing and calling. 'Hello? *Hello?*'

Ray slapped a hand to her forehead. '*Christ*,' she said.

'Ray, I can *see you* in there. Can I just ask you something quickly please?'

Ray rolled her eyes. Several nurses laughed or tutted, before one got up and drew the curtain.

'Hey!' Hodi yelled. 'That's not very nice!'

Another nurse stood up from a desk and opened the door. I could hear her telling Hodi that Ray was busy.

'But she's always busy!' Hodi replied.

'Step back please,' the nurse was saying to him. 'Move your foot.'

Ray leant forward in her chair and called to him. 'Not *now*, Hodi, I'll come to you in *one* minute.'

The nurse shut the door and let out a long breath.

'*One minute*,' we could hear Hodi saying. 'Always *one* minute. Then nothing . . .'

Twenty minutes passed, and Ray was on the phone.

'Raaay! Raaay! Can I just ask you *one* thing? *Pleeease.*'

Ray rolled her eyes, apologized to the receiver and then, cupping her hand over the end, leant towards a nurse on a nearby chair. 'Would you do me a favour?' she said. 'Can you just give him 4mg of lorazepam? He's driving me *nuts*.'

A little while later, Hodi reappeared back outside the office. His eyes were noticeably heavy, his features drooping. His trademark grin absent.

'Caall myy ddaadd!' he slurred heavily through the glass booth, the words rolling around on his lethargic tongue. 'Youu haave givenn mme a drrug wittthouut his perrrmission!'

THE TREATMENT ROOM

I felt myself look sharply at Ray. 'What have you given him?' I asked, feeling the words stick in my throat.

Ray clicked her pen and picked up the phone receiver. 'It's a sedative,' she said calmly. 'He needs to sleep, he hasn't slept in twenty-four hours.'

My mind was spinning. 'You . . . want him to sleep in the daytime?'

'Yes,' Ray said, turning to look at Hodi through the glass. 'You need to go to sleep!' she hollered. 'You'll feel much better!' She turned to the phone again and began punching at the numbers. 'It would be *great* if he slept in the daytime,' she said into the receiver.

I watched Hodi slope back to his bedroom, shock making me light-headed. *Had that really just happened?*

*

Treatment in psychiatry exists in shades of grey. It's medication acting on a person's body and mind in multiple imprecise and unclear ways. As a result, the language around drug effects appears to bewilder both staff and patients. Is sedation part of the treatment, or a side effect? Should these drugs be prescribed to control behaviour or just for treatment, and is there a difference between the two? Is it acceptable to damage the body through treating the mind?

*

The next morning, I was assigned to work in the treatment room. A bright white cube with no windows, lined with shelves of medical paraphernalia and locked mini-fridges full of pharmaceutical boxes. In the door was a shuttered hatch which could be pulled up and down and locked, with a double-sided ledge to lean across.

Such rooms have notorious connotations within our psyche and consequently within our art. Countless films, books and TV series have depicted them as the epicentre of cold, clinical conduct, devoid of empathy. I could see why. The sterility of the room felt merciless and unrelenting. A uniformity so far removed from the haphazard contours and colours of nature it seemed to exemplify a kind of madness of its own. But treatment is meant to connote compassion; from one human to another, from ourselves to our bodies. Perhaps it is this contradiction which feels frightening.

When I stepped into the room, I thought of the famous psychological experiment Still Face conducted in 1975 by Dr Edward Tronick. In it, a mother sits with her baby and plays normally. Then she turns round, rearranges her face into a blank expression, and looks back at her child. At first the baby watches her, unperturbed. Then it tries to get the warm reaction it had expected by pointing, smiling. When this is met with blankness, the baby starts to become distressed; rocking, looking away, screeching, before finally sobbing. Research tells us that when a child receives a continuous unempathetic reaction beyond this point, it goes into emotional shutdown to protect itself. It disassociates from its pain and sadness due to not having been 'met' psychologically. It too becomes blank – empty.

The treatment room has come to embody something

indescribable. It is a human face without expression. It is a void, echoing nothing.

Saul was awake. He found me hovering outside the treatment room and tapped me on the shoulder.

'Oi,' he said, 'you look sick.' He frowned at me.

'Oh, I . . . thanks,' I replied, feeling exposed.

Saul put his hand in the back pocket of his jeans and pulled out a curled book. 'Guess what?' he said. 'See this? I didn't even know there were books in this shithole!' He was grinning. 'What d'you know? Books!'

He pointed at a nurse who was coming out of the office and pretended to spit at her. 'That woman tried to give me zopiclone before she could be fucked to go find the library for me last night. *Books* help me sleep! They can shove their sedative up their fuckin' arses. I'm already addicted to that other shit they give me.'

A broad-shouldered nurse in a short-sleeved shirt pushed open the door, his face puckered with irritation. He muttered something. Saul and I watched as he went to stand in front of the reception desk and peered into the beehive behind it.

'Hello?' he said, snapping his fingers to get someone's attention. 'Is there a pen in there?'

A nurse opened the glass door. 'Thanks *so much* for today, Leon,' she said, smiling. 'You're our hero.'

Leon looked back at her indifferently. 'Fine. Fine.' He waved his hand. 'Is there a pen in there?'

The nurse pointed at the biro attached to the Patient Leave clipboard, where patients permitted short stints outside with a member of staff signed themselves in and out. 'There's one,' she said, gesturing.

Leon grunted. 'I'm not touching the patient pen,' he said.

Saul leant towards me. 'Leon works on PICU,' he whispered. 'I spent one week there and I'll tell you – if the devil himself was on that ward, I'd feel sorry for him.'

Leon walked down the corridor, having been given another pen. He looked at me, then at Saul, then back at me.

'Hi,' he said. 'Apparently you're with me for medication round.'

The Psychiatric Intensive Care Unit, or PICU, is where patients deemed violent or highly volatile are first taken to be treated. These wards tend to be smaller, with higher staffing levels, heftier locks and security doors, more harm-restrictive furnishings and easier-to-access 'de-escalation rooms'. Patients can be removed from the communal environment, usually by restraint, and locked inside these seclusion areas to 'calm down'.

The two de-escalation rooms in our building were approximately three metres square. They had heavy security doors and observation mirrors for staff to monitor the patient. Each room was devoid of fixtures and fittings which could be damaged, used for self-harm or as 'ligature' points – places to hang yourself – and had limited ventilation and no external light. The walls and floor were lined with sky-blue padding, and there was a single foam mattress in the corner. To me, these seclusion rooms were the stuff of nightmares.

I asked Leon why he was on our ward today.

'Staff shortages,' he said. '*Again*. And I've already worked more than sixty hours this week.'

'Wow.' I was taken aback. 'Does that happen a lot?'

Leon wasn't looking at me as he moved about the treatment room, gathering water cups and paper pill-pots. 'I *told* them I'm not coming down here, this isn't my job,' he said, taking a bundle of keys from his pocket and unlocking the shutter in the hatch. He pushed it open and it clattered noisily.

As we waited for the first patient, I moved about the room checking the names off a list I'd been given, noticing that I felt oddly sure of myself. Here my task as a nurse was clear: count out tablets, check dates, tick charts. While in the rest of the ward the job was opaque. Alongside the admin and practicalities, was it our job to *talk* to patients? And if so, in what way, for how long, and did we have the training to do so? I thought back to the three-hour 'foundation level' training we'd been given at university titled 'How to Talk to People in Distress', followed swiftly by a completion certificate given to all participants, regardless of their level of enthusiasm or involvement. The perfunctory skills imparted, such as listening affirmations, open questions and non-threatening body language, had left me baffled – surely that can't be all we're given before going into practice? I wondered if this was partly what led nurses to cluster in the office or the beehive, concealing themselves for hours. Interaction with patients was psychologically challenging and often distressing, requiring an energy and skill set the majority of us lacked.

I emptied four coloured pills into a paper pot and filled a glass of water, putting them both in front of Leon.

'But I make over forty thousand a year, you know,' he said, raising his eyebrows.

I stood, unsure what to say to this unexpected admission. 'That's . . . great,' I managed.

'It's a lot of money,' he clarified. 'You see, people like me take jobs on wards because the money's better, and because we're tougher people. The snowflakes mostly go work in the community because they can't take it. But PICU, that's a piece of cake for me. I used to be a mental health nurse in my country, so.'

He paused and leant back against the counter.

'What was it like there?' I asked, curious.

'*Well.*' He paused, seemingly for effect. 'When I was working there I thought it was fine. But then I came over here and it's so, so much better. Everything works and is properly sterile. Patients can get some outside time, you know. They have a TV and things like that. I thought, wow, this is so good! These patients don't know how lucky they are.'

I took this in, the quandary catching me off guard. I hadn't considered that to some people a comparison could be made casting this ward in a favourable light. I watched Leon, his eyes having taken on the unfocused sheen of reminiscence.

'That's interesting,' I replied.

Leon shook himself back into the room. He smiled. 'But I like the *action*,' he continued. 'People who work on wards like ACTION. You know? Ac-tion. And it's different all the time, very flexi. It's exciting, and yeah, it's hard too. You have to be strong.'

I turned from him and busied myself with moving cups around as he leant out of the hatch and bellowed Saul's name.

A few minutes passed before Saul moved into the frame. He looked down at the pills. My stomach told me something was wrong. Some kind of shame made me turn away.

'Hmm,' Saul said, looking steadily at Leon. He leant with all his weight on the counter, rubbed at one of his eyes and smiled thinly. 'Well, hello hello hello again.'

Leon ignored him and pushed the paper cup of tablets closer to Saul's arm.

Saul picked it up and tipped the coloured pills into the palm of his hand. He studied them.

'Right . . .' he said. 'You know, I don't even know what these pills *are*.'

Leon turned sharply and began opening another bottle, the muscles in his forearm flexing.

'I mean, seriously,' Saul tried again. 'What *are* these? I've been a guinea pig for years!'

Leon turned back abruptly, and for a moment I thought he was going to swipe the bottles off the hatch. Saul's eyes widened.

'Yes, *you do know* what they are, Saul!' he hissed. 'Most of them are for your physical health. Take them quickly, please, we don't have for ever.'

Saul sighed and knocked back the tablets, draining the glass of water noisily. He curtseyed elaborately before moving off to make space for the next patient.

As patients followed suit, filtering up to the hatch one by one, I asked Leon about PICU. The question seemed to calm him, his shoulders dropping.

'You see, you students are scared of PICU, but it's easier up there. Patients don't mess around like they do on this ward, they don't try and refuse their medication, because they know we'll just give them an injection. So, it's calmer, you know? It's not as scary as everyone thinks.'

I watched Leon hand a pill-pot to another patient more gently now. The word 'injection' swimming in my head.

'You . . . enjoy working there?' I asked, the words forming slowly.

'Yeah,' he said confidently, 'I do. I can take you up there, no problem.'

'Ah,' I heard myself say. 'Maybe.'

Leon laughed. 'Scared, huh? *See.*'

I turned from him. 'Something like that.'

A patient leant in through the hatch and waved his arm at us. 'You done chatting?' he said.

Leon spun round. 'Go back!' he yelled. 'Get out of the hatch!'

The patient laughed, took his paper cup off the counter and began walking away with it.

Leon leant with all his weight on the shelf. 'Come back here and take it where I can see you!' he shouted after him.

The man crept back and gulped down the pills. 'Dah-da!' he said.

Leon turned back to me. 'Piss-taker.' He shook his head. 'I'm not saying stuff doesn't happen there,' he continued, 'it does. My colleague got punched in the face last week by some patient. I've had a couple of sprained wrists. You heard about the guy with the fork?'

The patient-with-the-fork story had floated around the Acute Ward as well as my class at uni, its reliability unquestioned. It was shared with the fervour of an allegory, yet no one seemed to know how to interpret its significance beyond instilling an omnipresent fear. The tale was one of a patient on a PICU who had been given metal cutlery instead of wood.

Soon after, he had slammed the fork into his left eye, before skewering the palm of a nurse who'd come to stop him.

'Yeah, you see?' Leon was saying. '*Exactly*.'

There was a pause as we both, perhaps, contemplated the meaning behind his words.

Leon was wagging his finger, scolding the air. 'And I don't like being dragged down here,' he growled. 'This isn't my job. These patients get away with anything they want . . . asking what *this* is, what *that* is. What the *fuck*.'

I watched him clear away the medicine bottles silently before jerking at the hatch shutter and locking it.

'I think,' I began tentatively, unsure what I was going to say. 'I think I would ask what my medication was too if I was here. It seems to change a lot, you know?'

Leon looked at me, his mouth pulled away from his nose as if he'd smelt something repulsive. 'Well, I'd trust the *professionals*,' he said.

'Would you?' I continued. 'You think you wouldn't ask questions about your treatment if you were a patient on this ward?'

He turned away, his wide shoulders a barricade between us. Then his voice began, low and clipped: 'I'd never do anything that meant I'd *be* a patient here, so I don't have to worry about that.'

Throughout the day, Leon's frustration built. His movements becoming more condensed, his voice sharp. By the time evening medication was due, he was mumbling angrily to himself and slamming pill bottles on to the countertop.

I was outside the day area, having been asked to monitor

the line of patients as they filed up to Leon's treatment hatch. I was relieved to be watching from this side of the counter. Having been unable to decipher the fuel behind his contempt for the people he was nursing, I'd felt my own rage rising and worried I was going to lose my composure – something I couldn't afford to do as a student. These were my *teachers*, the people who could pass or fail me.

Hodi was last in the dinner queue in the day area. He adjusted his baseball cap as he waited to be served his dessert. 'Cheers mate,' he said to the health care assistant, taking the bowl of cake and custard from the counter and walking out of the room. Once in the hall, Hodi made his way over to the treatment hatch. I watched him standing in line for a few minutes, jiggling from side to side, before speaking loudly over the heads of two patients waiting in front of him.

'Yo!' he called to Leon. 'Can I just have some paracetamol?'

Leon stiffened, his head rising slowly to look Hodi in the eye, before fixing on the bowl of food in his right hand. 'You can't walk around with that!' he yelled. 'Go and sit down and stop getting in everyone's way!'

Hodi's head and neck withdrew into his shoulders. Several patients looked up at him, waiting for a reaction. Noticing them, he pushed his chest forward purposefully.

'Hey! I just want a paracetamol! Then I'll eat this. What are you shouting at me for?'

Leon leant further forward out of the hatch, his voice low this time. 'Go and do as you're told, or I'll give you something *other* than paracetamol.'

A health care assistant, sensing the tension, approached swiftly and attempted to take hold of Hodi's waist and pull him away. In his shock, he momentarily let his body follow hers, then turned back, pulling his torso away, and shouted with force, 'What? Is that a *threat*? Yeah? I have rights, you dickhead! I'm not taking anything you give me!'

Leon smirked, his face calm. 'You know you'll *have* to take it if you get angry.'

The bowl in Hodi's hand fell to the floor, shattering on impact. Custard smeared in spider-like veins across the pale blue laminate. Before I knew it Hodi was pushing his way through the other men, launching his body towards Leon. Two nurses emerged in the hallway, surveying the danger, their bodies sharp, hands on their alarms. They started running.

'Grab him!' Leon shouted. 'Take him to seclusion!'

In desperation, I yelled Hodi's name. I asked him to *wait*, to *stop*. In the confusion he let me take his arm and steer him up the hallway, away from the commotion. We stopped some metres away, both breathing heavily.

'What . . . what's his problem, man?' he shouted at me, looking back towards Leon.

'He's stressed, Hodi!' My voice came out too loudly. 'He . . . shouldn't have said that . . . just . . . let it go, please!' My body was pulsing with anger and fear, but desperation made me plead. '*Don't*, Hodi. Just walk away. You know what will happen if you don't . . . *please*.'

Hodi looked at me and jerked his cap down over his eyes, his arms crossing his body awkwardly. 'That cunt better not come anywhere near me . . . just *watch* if he does.' Stiffly, he skulked away, back into the day area, where he stood silently at the counter, waiting for another dessert.

*

I avoided speaking to any of the staff for hours. My head was whirring like a mechanical toy, my body moving as if suspended above the ground. Staff passed me in the corridors, moving from room to room, continuing their duties. Yet now, they appeared conspiratorial. They broke eye contact too soon, huddled in groups and spoke in whispers.

Someone tapped my shoulder. I spun round.

Fuad – the nurse I'd met when Irene left with the ambassador.

'Are you OK?' he asked, inspecting me. Up close his face looked as worn and soft as old leather.

'I'm OK.' I breathed. 'I'm . . . Thanks for asking.'

I didn't feel OK; my limbs didn't feel like my own. Fuad continued to peer at me.

'That wasn't a good scene,' he said gently. 'Well done for stepping in when you did.' His eyes squinted with concern. 'Not a good scene at all.'

'I guess,' I began, thoughts rushing from me. 'I mean, how can you let that *happen* here?' I heard the anger in my voice, my legs starting to shake with adrenalin again.

Fuad's body appeared to solidify and he looked at the floor, nodding in short, sharp little nods. 'Yeah, yeah. He is . . . I mean, he is not normally on this ward and, well, we have a problem with staffing, and I . . . I can't make an excuse for him, or anyone.'

I was suddenly embarrassed. I wasn't helping anybody by being angry with this man. My eyes pricked with tears.

'I'm sorry. I just mean . . . I'm just shocked.'

'No, it's OK. Really.' Fuad clasped his arms around his chest. 'It's all true what you said. I'm actually thinking of going to work on this therapeutic ward. To get out of here, you know? It's called The Garden. Have you heard of it? It's the only one of its kind in the NHS in this city. It's meant to be really great, really different. I was going to go there a while ago but—'

'The Garden?'

'Yeah. I've heard that it's, well, it's more of a community with lots of activities, therapy, groups. I've just heard, I don't know. I haven't seen it.'

Another nurse called to us from across the hallway – there was a meeting starting. Fuad smiled weakly.

'Try not to . . . worry,' he said.

Worry? I thought. The word seemed insubstantial.

We walked together to the beehive, and I felt myself mirroring him. It felt calming, for once, to be in step with someone. I'd been on placement for over a month and this was the first time I'd experienced a sense of camaraderie.

Fuad opened the door and greeted another nurse warmly. Watching him, I wondered if, after so many years assimilating into this place, he truly believed that doing things differently was possible.

The beehive was already full, with staff resting on surfaces and chatting animatedly. The health care assistant from the fight was mid-flow.

'And then he said, "Say that again to my face!" and I tried to grab him, you know, so I could de-escalate him. But he smashed his food on the floor . . .'

A nurse with purple hair was laughing. '*Jesus*, that kid! Did it work?'

'What?'

'The de-escalation!'

'Oh, well.' The health care assistant grinned. 'You know how that boy is.'

'Honestly.' The nurse chuckled again and leant over to take a chocolate biscuit from the desk. 'I would have just given him a rapid tranq.'

The health care assistant started laughing. 'Oh, don't get me wrong,' she said, 'I'm all about a good injection, but I don't mind doing a bit of de-escalation every so often.'

I looked at Fuad shrunken in his chair, his mind elsewhere.

Two days later I joined the weekly patient evaluation meeting. During these meetings, Dr Oxley reviewed prescriptions and treatment plans through a series of questions levelled at the nurse-in-charge about each patient's 'presentation'.

I sat between three junior nurses and across from the nurse-in-charge as the doctor called out the first patient's name. I pictured them in my mind, standing still in a blank room, their physique fuzzy, as if they were waiting for us to define them.

As I listened to the nurse's descriptions, I felt the room grow more suffocating. The outlines didn't join up. The narratives seemed skewed. The nurse-in-charge had been given so much disjointed information from the threadbare staff and agency workers on awkward shift rotations that what she was saying about patients was barely intelligible, let alone illuminating. There was no consistency to the depictions of concern or improvement, no reliability or accuracy to the vital information passed between nurse and consultant.

No one is actually talking to the patients, I thought.

'OK, fine.' Dr Oxley was scratching a sentence through with a green pen. 'We'll just up his sertraline and see how that goes. Next. Hodi? I heard there was an incident?'

Today's nurse-in-charge hadn't been on the ward that day. She began to tell another story, one I didn't recognize. One in which Hodi starred as the aggressor.

Dr Oxley's eyebrows furrowed as he listened, his forehead creasing. He studied Hodi's medication chart.

'Right, well, what to do with *this* guy?' His lips puckered. 'We could . . . up his lorazepam. Yes, it seems he's still too agitated.'

'Erm . . .'

Suddenly, I was speaking. Everyone in the room turned to look at me. I felt my cheeks flush with blood.

'I was there. I mean . . . I saw it. I was with Hodi.'

How to word this without sounding like I was calling the nurse-in-charge a liar? Without naming everyone else in the room as complicit?

I was sat bolt upright, my eyes fixed on the doctor. He looked right back at me.

No one spoke. I shifted in my chair.

'It's actually . . . I mean, how it happened was . . . I think Leon was very stressed, having a stressful day, and Hodi brought food into the hallway, and was asking for paracetamol, but . . . he wasn't being very patient really, and Leon sort of provoked him – by accident – and Hodi reacted.'

My cheeks were burning. I could see myself through Dr Oxley's eyes: mumbling, rouged, unprofessional.

'So,' he said, his eyes still on me, 'he might have been

provoked?' He looked to the other faces in the room. 'But he still reacted aggressively? Was he able to be de-escalated?'

A nurse who had been present at the incident between Leon and Hodi spoke up for the first time. 'Yes,' she said, 'he was de-escalated. He didn't need a rapid tranq.'

There was a moment of silence. The nurse-in-charge was flipping her sheet of notes back and forth and shaking her head. 'Well, I'd been told something different for some reason.'

Dr Oxley stared at the medication chart in front of him, his right thumb digging at the corner of a fingernail.

'Fine, fine. Let's just leave his medication for now then and see how the week goes.'

The next day I trawled through patient files for hours, reading the daily notes written by staff which are used to determine treatment reviews and ongoing sectioning. I pored over recent entries for patients I'd spent time with. One psychology report documented that Saul was *still very delusional as he continues to express the belief that his life is being controlled by doctors through the use of medication, and is overly preoccupied with professionals involved in his case*. I noted this down, bewildered by their proclamation that a belief so close to Saul's actual reality was instead a psychotic delusion.

I then came across a note written the previous day. *Hodi*, it said, *is still thought disordered today. He has continued laughing inappropriately to himself and it's likely he's hearing voices.* I looked at the time of the note. I had been with Hodi most of yesterday afternoon and thought back to our conversations.

He had been completely rational and stable; I couldn't think of one single concern about his conduct.

Buzzing with frustration, I found the author of the entry organizing a fridge in the treatment room. I poked my head through the hatch.

'Can I ask what you were referring to with this incident?' I said, handing her the printed version of her note.

The nurse looked confused.

'I'm just trying to understand his diagnosis,' I offered.

The nurse nodded and thought for a moment. She told me she'd seen him coming out of the day area, laughing to himself. *I remember this*, I thought. We'd just been laughing together about a TV programme. Someone had made a joke. It had been funny. He'd walked out of the room, still laughing. I told the nurse this.

'Oh,' she said, her face impassive.

I looked at her, wanting more than this as acknowledgement.

'*OK*,' she said, tucking a strand of hair behind her ear.

I made a mental note to check if she amended the file.

A few days later, it remained unchanged.

For several days, the ward was calm. Staff came and went, patients woke and slept and took their medication. A strange, soporific rhythm ensued, yet for me it remained tinged with the sharp threat of aggression.

While I was on leave over the weekend, a new patient, Bertie, arrived. On the Monday I found him wandering from room to room, confused and close to tears. As he walked, his feet fumbled over each other, his long dreadlocked hair bouncing around his arms, his hands gripping multiple items of clothing, a toothbrush, a pen, a bag, a battered straw hat. He often lost balance, using furniture or walls to prop against. Then he would stand stock-still, stare as if trying to penetrate the brick, and tell you he had forgotten what he was going to do. Bertie's words were incomprehensibly slurred and troubling to follow. His sentences began with gusto before trailing off like a mechanism winding down.

That afternoon, I found Fuad and asked him about Bertie's sedation.

'Oh.' He paused.

I had come to recognize his nervous features when I approached, suddenly conscious of my own pensive expression, pen in hand, tatty notepad at the ready.

'He's been prescribed lorazepam – the benzodiazepine – four times daily,' Fuad explained.

He was midway through his fifteen-minute checks on patients deemed high-risk to themselves. This involved peeking into rooms to check each person was moving, waiting for the rise and fall of their chest, before ticking through their name on a clipboard. I walked beside him as I noted this down.

'As a sedative, or for anxiety? I mean, was he . . .' I hesitated. 'Was he violent when he came in?'

Fuad stopped outside the day area and, seeing a man's back hunched on the sofa, ticked off another name.

'He, well, I think he was pretty agitated, yeah. He was angry at being brought in, something about pushing someone into a wall. The police took him in on Section 136.'

'Oh. That's a twenty-four-hour section, right?'

'Yeah. Police can detain someone if they think they've got a mental disorder. But the lorazepam, I . . . think it's too much, really. *Way* too much.' He looked off into the distance, no longer addressing me. 'He can barely stand up or remember his name half the time. I've said that lots of times in handover. I've told Dr Oxley.'

I was relieved by Fuad's annoyance; it made me feel safe – the sturdiness of solidarity.

'He fell over again this morning,' I said. 'Did you know? I'm worried he's going to hit his head.'

Fuad roused from inertness and began moving down the hallway again. He opened a bedroom door with his free hand and raised a palm towards the prostrate man on the bed. The man raised his hand silently in response. Tick.

'And benzodiazepines are addictive,' he said. 'Which is complicated, and tricky . . . very difficult to get off them, you know.'

I continued, feeling hopeful, 'And he's not aggressive at all.'

'And he's falling all over the place.'

'Yeah.'

Fuad stopped walking. I noticed he was clicking the pen in his fist repetitively.

'I'll bring it up with Dr Oxley again,' he said. 'It needs to be brought up again.'

Together, Fuad and I wrote two notes in Bertie's file, documenting our concerns and requesting that his benzodiazepine be reduced. Fuad shared his apprehensions in a nursing meeting and requested to speak to the consultant. Five days went by with no changes made to his dosage.

Bertie passed out while shaving, his unconscious face falling into a sink of water.

He was revived.

A hurried meeting was called: if he hadn't been closely monitored due to the razor, he wouldn't be alive. Dr Oxley reduced his lorazepam swiftly, to three times and then two times daily. In the succeeding days, Bertie was visibly more stable on his feet and coherent in his thoughts.

Over a week passed on the new medication regime. It was morning, and I joined another handover, this time in the cramped office. The room was bathed in white from the ceiling strip, and the row of old computers were humming. The chatter around me was upbeat, and I heard several of the nurses remark that Bertie was 'so much better' and 'getting so well'. I turned towards them, looking at each of their faces. I was looking for something I couldn't pinpoint, watching their mouths move, their skin stretch about their features. No one mentioned the medication change. I could feel an artery throbbing in my neck.

'By *well*,' my mouth began, 'do you mean that he's less sedated because his lorazepam was reduced after the sink incident?'

There was silence.

'Perhaps,' responded a nurse carefully. 'But probably he's just getting better from his illness.'

I felt myself squinting. The artery pounded.

'By *better*, do you mean more coherent?' I was dumbstruck – this was a medical professional's assessment.

The nurse cleared his throat and looked at me with heavy eyelids, his features flaccid. 'The drugs sort out the biology problems in the brain,' he said confidently, then turned back to his sheet of notes. 'Shall we start?' he asked the room.

I left that meeting as evenly as I could. I needed to be outside. To be anywhere else. But, as always, there was another meeting to attend, and I only had a few minutes. I slipped into the staff room, a depressingly characterless room with two matching sofas, a microwave, a sink and a framed poster of Van Gogh's *Sunflowers*. I leant against the wall, and watched an ambulance pass slowly by the window. I closed my eyes.

Behind me, I heard the door open.

'Hey!'

I turned to see a familiar ruddy-cheeked, yellow-bearded face smiling at me.

'Alex!' I said loudly. 'What are you doing here?'

'Placement buddies,' he announced with a grin, his lanyard shining against his black hoodie.

'You're on my ward?'

'Yup!' he said. 'Here I am.'

Behind him, a nurse stopped. 'If you're not on break yet,' she said, 'could you come out of here, please?'

I apologized, and Alex and I left the room, feeling like naughty teenagers.

'I'm meant to sign in,' Alex whispered, 'but I couldn't see anyone in the office.'

'Oh,' I said. 'I'll let you in.'

After fumbling with the office lock for a minute, we walked in together, each bolstered by the presence of the other. In the corner of the room a grey-haired psychiatrist I'd not seen before in a tweed coat sat flanked by two trainees. He held up his hand to us in greeting.

'Oh, sorry to interrupt,' I said, dipping my head automatically.

'*My* apologies,' he replied theatrically. 'We'll be finished and out in one minute. No need to go anywhere.'

Alex swivelled a chair and flopped on to it, swinging back and forth. There was something enviable, I thought, in his heavy-limbed indiscretion. *Here I am*, his body seemed to say to the space around it. *Make way.*

'OK.' I perched on an adjacent chair. 'Thank you.'

The psychiatrist leant in to his students. 'So really,' he said, 'to answer your question about the sexual abuse she experienced – we can't *assume* this had a significant impact on her. It could be relevant, or it could not be. You have to be careful making *tenuous* links.'

One of the young men flushed and looked at his feet.

'We're only in contact with people who need *help* after a sexual assault or abuse,' he continued. 'Not the people who are *just fine* and *get on* with it. Which is many.'

The other trainee, in a pressed white shirt and suit jacket, waved a fountain pen. 'Would you also think it's worth treating her for suspected ADHD?'

The psychiatrist leant back in his chair and folded his arms above his distended stomach. 'Yes. ADHD and personality disorder. I'd also note that vegetarianism in teenage girls is often indicative of an eating disorder in the making.'

I felt my eyes widen. Alex stopped his rotation.

The trainees noted this down on their pads as the psychiatrist got to his feet. They bobbed up in unison.

'All *yours*, ladies and gentlemen,' the psychiatrist said to us, taking a handkerchief from his top pocket and dabbing at his nose. 'Let's get a cup of tea, chaps.'

We watched them trail out and close the door behind them.

'So,' Alex said, looking towards the door, 'what's going on in *this* place? Lots of public-schooled doctors?'

I laughed, realizing how much I'd missed laughing.

'Did he actually just say that?' I said, my cheeks tight.

'Wow! Yeah, he definitely did. Is he the regular consultant here?'

'I've never seen him before, thankfully.'

Alex shook his head. 'Unlucky for the poor patient they've just seen.' He paused. 'I've been thinking... if we make everything a *medical* problem, then it's no longer a social problem.' He looked up at me. 'So, nothing needs to be addressed: just prescribe a pill and move on. The medical world doesn't really know what to do with distress, so we drug the person, because that's what medics are taught to do.'

'Alex,' I said, 'thank God you're here.'

'Them's the facts,' he said, smiling. 'Can't mince the facts.'

'But honestly...' I breathed out heavily. 'I think I'm starting to lose my—'

'Nope,' he interrupted. 'Not allowed. None of that on my watch.'

Alex spun on his chair again, his legs lifted from the floor. He looked like a happy child. It was surreal to see him here, in this place.

'I'm so glad you're here,' I repeated.

'Oh.' He looked serious. 'I'm only here for the day apparently.'

'What?' I felt like the air had been sucked out of me. 'Just today?'

'Yeah, day trip. Then I go back to the forensic secure ward,' he replied. 'It's brutal there, for sure. Though I might be back later.'

There was a knock on the door. We both looked towards it.

A nurse with waxy spiked hair opened it wide. He smiled at us.

'I'm Gabe,' he said. 'I'm giving an introduction to ECT now.' He looked from Alex to me slowly, watching for our reaction. 'You want to come along?'

My only experience with electro-convulsive therapy was hearing a patient brought on to the ward and beg the staff around her, '*Please* don't give me ECT again. It was awful . . . awful. I lost my brain.'

The memory of her words sent a shiver through me.

As Alex and I followed Gabe to the ECT Suite, I thought back to the conflicting articles I'd read about electro-convulsive therapy. Despite some practitioners and patients giving weighty exaltations to its outcomes, there were equally loud protestations over its significant harm. Those who called it torture, enforced brain damage. I couldn't deny that I felt biased; I didn't like the idea one bit and couldn't imagine myself ever administering it to someone. Even walking past the sign outside the building made me uneasy. *What is it that concerns me so much?* Before my training started I hadn't realized ECT was still being used in psychiatry. For something so physically as well as psychologically intrusive, so potentially permanent, to be *forced* on anyone felt morally dubious. Even the suggestion that it caused brain damage was enough to outweigh any potential benefit for me, and the fact it could be used on someone before they were able to decide for themselves overstepped a line I didn't feel willing to cross. But I could be open-minded. Couldn't I?

'This is an excellent facility, world class. Not every hospital has one.' Gabe was beaming as he walked us down to the suite. 'So, we're very lucky.'

Alex raised an eyebrow at me.

'What type of patients tend to use it?' he asked Gabe, putting his hands into the pouch of his hoodie.

'Oh.' Gabe moved towards him, enlivened by the engagement. 'We have one patient who comes back here all the time, says it's the only thing that works for her. It's for the depressed mainly. And the treatment-resistant.' He tugged at the skin on his neck.

'Right,' I replied involuntarily. I could hear the sarcasm in my voice. 'And how does it actually work?'

Gabe's face seemed to flatten with irritation. It wasn't the question he'd wanted. 'Well, it . . . resets the brain.'

*

Despite being in use for over eighty years, what ECT does to the brain and body is still not understood. Yet around 2,500 ECT treatments are carried out each year in England, with approximately 58 per cent of patients being over the age of sixty, and 67 per cent being female.

Various theories have been proposed over the years and, as with much treatment in psychiatry, practitioners disseminate their preferred theory, or give poorly understood, generic information to patients. One dominant theory is that ECT causes damage to the brain cells which results in temporary euphoria, followed by emotional blunting and memory loss. In fact, studies have found that between 12 and 55 per cent of people given ECT suffer long-lasting or permanent brain damage resulting in memory difficulties.

Whether or not this effect is deemed a beneficial treatment and the negative effects acceptable seems to depend on who is evaluating and recording 'improvements'. For example, if a person is unable to remember parts of their life after ECT, some of which caused them distress, a doctor may consider their subsequent reduced distress about these experiences to be a 'success'. Whereas the person given the ECT may consider their memory loss frightening or detrimental, as in the case of the patient I'd overheard on our ward. The desired outcome of ECT remains intangible.

Yet despite documented effects as serious as brain damage, a person can still be given ECT without consent if a psychiatrist believes it could alleviate their suffering, or prevent them from behaving violently towards themselves or others. The patient and their family will not be able to weigh the risks up first.

*

When we arrived at the suite there were other student nurses in the waiting area. Everyone was sat with a cup of tea, and a packet of chocolate digestives was being passed around. Gabe disappeared briefly, and after some minutes reappeared again. He stepped into the room as if it was his stage, looking carefully at each of our faces and rubbing his hands together excitedly.

'So!' he began. 'My bet is that most of you are thinking about *One Flew Over the Cuckoo's Nest*.'

Some of the students nodded and smiled awkwardly.

'Well, let me start by saying that those were *unregulated* doses used as punishment. That's not what we do here.'

A young, slight woman put up her hand. 'Is there a dominant theory about how it works?' she asked.

Gabe wiped his forehead and smiled. He'd had some time to prepare for this question in the wings. 'Thank you for your enquiry. Well, no one knows *exactly* how it works, but I can tell you that it does, it really does. And it's life-saving!'

I looked around at the faces in the room, trying to guess their thoughts. This was hardly a satisfactory answer. Was anyone going to question him further?

'For example,' Gabe continued, 'we have a patient who comes in once a week who doesn't eat or drink at all. After ECT she stuffs her face with biscuits.' He smiled.

A few people tittered into the silence.

'No, but really. What I'm saying is, they suddenly start eating, straight after. It's quite something.' He paused, sensing he was losing the crowd. 'Last week,' he pressed on, 'a patient of ours had her one hundred and twentieth ECT treatment and she couldn't be happier. Nothing else was working for her!'

I put my hand up. A look of distaste passed over his face.

'What about memory loss?' I asked, feeling the grip of adrenalin.

'Or brain damage?' Alex stepped forward beside me.

'Nope,' Gabe said, looking slowly from me to Alex. '*None at all*. I don't know where people are getting that information.'

Gabe led us through two further waiting areas before stopping in a room containing a stark, wipeable bench-bed. On the table beside it was a box with multiple dials and wires that reminded me of a retro hi-fi. I found myself breathing out, relieved, realizing I'd expected a patient to be lying there.

Gabe strutted through us like a rooster among his hens.

'Voilà!' he said. 'The Therapy Unit.'

He laid a plastic mouthpiece on the bed. To my surprise, I found I could barely look at it.

'The patient bites down on this, to avoid any injuries to their teeth during the procedure.' He turned towards the hi-fi, picking up two wires with tiny discs on the end and holding them in the air. 'And these go on either side, or on the same side, of the brain. Depending on the patient, depending on the illness.'

I looked away. An insect pinged against the glass window.

'The anaesthetist will put them to sleep,' Gabe continued, 'administer a muscle relaxant to reduce the convulsions, and then the machine will send electrical pulses through the brain, causing what we refer to as a *controlled fit* for up to two minutes.'

I could feel my breathing quicken and turned to Alex, hoping his presence would steady me.

'Young lady.' Gabe's voice was louder now. He was pointing to a woman near me. 'Give me a current between one and a hundred to try out.'

The woman looked around her. There was a pause.

'Erm, eighty-five?' she offered.

Gabe clapped his hands together and rubbed them vigorously. 'Ooooh, she likes a BIG one!'

He turned towards the machine, his finger outstretched, and I felt myself holding my breath, as if, despite there being no actual patient in front of us, just witnessing the demonstration would implicate me in its use.

A student put up their hand.

'When can ECT be *forced* on a patient?' she asked.

Gabe turned back to his audience, putting his hands on his hips. He looked thoughtful for a moment. '*Well*,' he began, 'if two doctors feel it's needed and the person is too ill to consent. Actually, even if you're still waiting for the second doctor's opinion, and the first doctor feels it's immediately necessary, then under Section 62 it would be permissible to use force.'

He let this sink in.

'Remember,' he said, 'it's life-saving.'

'I've heard it's quite expensive?' another student said, chewing his fingernail. 'Is that correct?'

Gabe looked at him pointedly. 'Why do you ask that?'

The student looked embarrassed, his face flushing. 'Oh, sorry, I'm ... just curious really!' He laughed jauntily and looked around at us.

Gabe's muscles seemed to slacken. 'Oh well, in that case, yes, this is a private unit, ultimately, and we charge £400 per session to the NHS. This *is* a business at the end of the day, and we are doing very well thank you very much!'

*

What is it about mental illness that allows such extreme treatment? Perhaps confronting madness does something unique to us, shakes us to the core and – terrified – we seek to repress it, to control it. Aggressively, violently if we have to. An indescribable fear that feels ancient, primal; like our instinctual recoil from a snake, or disgust-fuelled jolt from something putrid.

3

The Hallway

We think of a hallway as a liminal space. A space where we are transitioning from one place to another; not yet there, but not where we began. There is a passivity to this depiction, casting hallways in an auxiliary role. But in hospitals they are throbbing with their own significance. A hallway can be an area of protest and discontent, a place to be acknowledged as someone needing, demanding. A place for people who refuse to fully inhabit the uncanny bedrooms and living areas that confine them to the role of 'patient'. The hallway impedes the enforced stagnancy; it is geared towards movement and tempts agency. Though, it is a labyrinthine offer. Blockaded at either end by weighty alarmed doors flanked by security guards, its proposition is an illusion.

Accident & Emergency is the nucleus of this liminality; it is the vital gateway between the outside world and the medical world, as well as this world and the afterworld. Hallways are where patients gather, wander, are treated. They are a continuation of every other space, enclosing the overspill of distress which cannot be confined behind flimsy curtains. In A&E, the tension of constant movement and unrelenting need encourages hasty, time-pressured assessments and decisions. People are one evaluation away from a diagnosis, a closed ward, a medication regime. It is where people become patients, leaving those hallways with a new, refracted lens through which to see themselves.

*

After two months on the Acute Ward, I was rotated for a short hiatus into emergency medicine. As students, we're encouraged both to embed ourselves within particular teams and experience the web of interconnecting routes into psychiatry. Placements were allocated via lottery, and emergency psychiatry – or 'psychiatric liaison' as it's known – was considered a golden ticket. Here, mental health nurses avoided the stagnation of the familiar; instead they wrestled with the rotation of new faces, new afflictions: from panic attacks to birth trauma to psychosis. It was said that you encountered more in A&E in a week than you would in a month on a ward.

The proposition of rotation felt both relieving and daunting to me. I would be temporarily back within the stitching of everyday reality among more familiar ailments, but A&E is also where the volatile and shocking accumulate. A place where we're forced to confront the precariousness of our daily functioning. A birth, death, life-shattering accident, near-miss – a lightning bolt into our mundane.

On my first day, I made my way past the sedentary ambulances snaking down the cul-de-sac and stood on the high street opposite the towering general hospital, watching people bustle in and out. My heart was beating steadily and I contemplated the shift of blood around my body. Though my mind felt strangely silent, calm. Perhaps, I wondered, my experiences on the ward had already hardened me with an armour that blunted emotion. Did I need my nerves to be raw to recognize pain or danger, to exist within the space between directive and action? Was I becoming more like the nurses around me, disassociating from the extremes of my daily reality in order to function within it?

The hospital's large glass doors slid open and I stepped in. It felt cavernous in comparison to the Acute Ward, the dejection bleached away by a stream of daylight. This hospital was mall-like, multi-floored and vibrated with activity. Each floor had a glass balcony circling the central hub of cafes, gift shops, receptions and waiting areas.

I passed through the clattering foyer and followed signs to Accident & Emergency, a giddiness spiking through me, as if I'd been plugged into the mains. My adrenalin had returned.

A&E was made up of ten curtained cubicles and two closed rooms around a central, bustling reception area. Doctors with phones pressed to their ears directed staff around with outstretched arms. The nurses confident and purposeful, harangued or frustrated. A mass of bodies and energy and movement.

A woman in an oversized flannel shirt and hoop earrings – distinguishable by her lanyard as a mental health nurse – smiled. She introduced herself as Afrah.

'You're with me today,' she said, warmly. 'I just need to let someone know I'll be with them in ten.' I could hear the tightness in her chest. 'They've been waiting a while.' She nodded to a nearby doctor before turning back to me. 'OK, let's drop your stuff and have a quick tour.'

We walked together to the office, Afrah slowing as she ascended the stairs. Her whole body emanating a creaking fatigue.

'You've been on an Acute Ward?'

I nodded.

'Well, you're used to intense then,' she said, 'but it's pretty relentless here.' She grasped at the handrail. 'Exciting, or a bit scary – depending on what you're into.' She made a little noise in place of a laugh. 'Though it's not the best day for you to arrive, to be honest. Not your fault, just that I've been on two doubles and spent the last God knows how many hours trying to find someone a bed that's not a thousand miles away. Anyway . . .' She trailed off and let out a shaky breath. '*Anyway.*'

I left my bag in the crowded office and Afrah pointed out the computers, break room and closed door to the psychiatrist's office, before we went back down to A&E. I followed her to a cubicle and she swept away the waxy blue curtain, the material clustering together chaotically. A dark-haired woman, so pale she looked grey, sat on a plastic chair next to the hospital bed, cradling her bandaged forearm in her lap. She peered at us from under her fringe.

Afrah grabbed a chair and dragged it opposite the woman, the metal legs squeaking across the floor. I propped myself awkwardly on the end of the bed.

The woman nodded at us. 'Don't think I've met you before,' she said vaguely. Her breath smelt sour, like old apples.

'No, we've not met. But you've seen some of my colleagues.' Afrah introduced us. 'So,' she continued, 'have you been drinking today, Leah?'

Leah blinked at her slowly, as if the question was beneath her. 'I had some drinks,' she said finally.

'OK,' Afrah said, scribbling on her notepad. 'Can you tell me what happened to your arm?'

'I already *told* someone,' she said wearily.

'Can you tell us?'

Leah stared at her arm in silence. 'I hate my arm,' she murmured, still looking away.

'What?'

'I *hate* my arm, it's done some fucked-up shit.'

'You hate your arm?' Afrah's pen hovered above the page.

'I think – as I told your colleague before – I'm just trying to *cope* with what happened. It doesn't leave me *alone*. It's terrible, terrible.'

'Your arm?'

'Me. *Me*.' Leah's face crumpled. 'I've done some terrible shit.'

Afrah paused.

'How did your arm go through the window, Leah?'

'What?'

'Did you punch the glass?'

Leah smiled thinly. 'No,' she said. 'I fell through it.'

Afrah looked blank. 'You *fell*?'

Leah continued to stare at her. 'Yes,' she said slowly. 'That's what I said.'

'Were you . . . *angry* with your arm?'

'Huh?'

'Angry?'

'I told you what happened,' Leah replied. 'I do hate this fucking arm though, served it right. I had to stab someone with it. They made me do it.'

Afrah paused again. A muscle twitched in her jaw.

'You're an ex-soldier, right? You were in Iraq?'

'Yeah. As I said, I'm trying to get the shit out of my head, but it doesn't go.'

'Can you tell me what's happening in your head?'

'All kinds of awful shit.' Leah wrapped her good arm around her body. 'You want to hear about it? I'd *love* to tell you, but I'm going to need more than five minutes.'

'Well, we haven't got a lot of time . . . sorry.' Afrah wrote down something I couldn't decipher. 'Can you tell me why you hurt yourself? Were you trying to kill yourself?'

Leah leant back in her chair. She looked at the floor. 'I – no. *No*. I don't know why I did it. I don't know why, OK? I just know that I feel pretty terrible.'

'Do you want to die?'

'No, not . . . really.'

'I'm confused that you don't know why you hurt yourself.'

'I told you, I feel like shit,' Leah said.

'But you weren't trying to kill yourself? You don't sound sure.'

'No. I mean yes, I'm sure.'

'Are you worried about yourself?'

'Yes, I mean . . . I'm not doing great, I guess.'

Afrah squinted and shifted the pen in her hand. 'What if I said you needed to be admitted to hospital?'

Leah frowned and shook her head. 'Why?'

'Because you're unwell.'

Leah's eyes spiked with tears and she shook her head again. 'Admission wouldn't help me. I've tried that. It's fucking awful.'

Afrah noted something down. 'Well,' she said, looking up from her notepad, 'I'm a mental health nurse, so I'll tell you if it would be helpful.'

Leah was quiet, and Afrah took an audible breath.

'I'm thinking about keeping you safe.'

'Well,' Leah responded. 'Can I *talk* to you then, or someone? Can I have some fucking therapy?'

Afrah fiddled with her pen again. 'Have you been referred for psychotherapy?'

'Yes. I'm on a waiting list that is seven hundred years long.'

'But you're on it.'

'That's what I said.'

Afrah nodded. 'Do you hear things or see things that aren't there?'

Pause. 'No.'

'Did a voice tell you to harm yourself?'

'Did I mention,' Leah said, looking at the ceiling, 'they won't give me therapy *before* I stop drinking?'

'Then you have to stop drinking, it's a maladaptive coping strategy.'

'Hah!' Leah clapped her hands together. 'Wow. Thanks.' She folded both arms across her.

Afrah was scribbling again. 'I'll refer you to—'

'I'm referred *everywhere*,' Leah said, rocking her head back.

'Did a voice tell you to harm yourself?' Afrah tried again.

'I don't think so.'

Afrah breathed out. She looked as though every drop of

energy had been squeezed out of her. 'OK,' she said. 'I'm going to speak to the doctor.'

Leah looked up. 'Great. If I could speak to them for more than five minutes too that would also be helpful.'

We left, drawing the curtain after us. Afrah walked behind the central reception desk and slumped on to an office chair. She yawned.

'I really, *really* need to get some coffee.'

I offered to find some.

'Wait, wait,' she said, flapping her hand at me. 'Here's Dr McCulloch.'

The familiar doctor, no longer in her Hawaiian print dress, was walking towards us, her reading glasses pushed up into her mess of grey hair. She smiled apologetically, as if she'd given us an unwanted task, and shook my hand, the string of beads around her neck bouncing.

She turned to Afrah. 'You've been to see Leah, then?'

'Yeah, she's back again.' Afrah sighed. 'I just don't *understand*. She doesn't seem to know why she does it. Seems very detached – it's weird. I'm not sure I believe what she's saying about not hearing things. She said something about hating her arm, which was a bit creepy.'

Dr McCulloch raised an eyebrow. 'Detached?'

'Hmm, I mean – psychotic depression perhaps? Her *insight* wasn't very good.'

Insight, I knew, was a psychiatric term that referred to a person's ability to recognize if they're mentally unwell. If it's decided that you 'lack insight', your ability to make decisions about your own treatment may be questioned, and the possibility that staff can usurp this responsibility rises.

I turned to Afrah, confused. 'Why do you say that?' I could feel myself frowning.

'Well, she didn't think she should go to hospital,' Afrah replied flatly.

'But, she said she was traumatized, she was asking for therapy.'

'Yeah, but they *all* say stuff like that. There's something else going on.'

Another nurse, overhearing, put her clipboard down on the desk. 'Leah's back, right?'

'Yeah.' Afrah shrugged. 'I just saw her.'

'Drunk and demanding therapy again?'

'Something like that.'

'Honestly,' the nurse said. 'Last time she came in she talked at me for an *hour*. Just a massive offload. I'm not so good at that stuff. Give me someone psychotic any day, just not someone who wants to *talk*.'

'I hear you,' Afrah said, rubbing at her eye. 'I'm sorry, I just don't have the bandwidth for it today. I'm done.'

Afrah checked the computer and scrolled through notes for a few minutes.

'She's on olanzapine already, and citalopram for the depression. Maybe she needs another antipsychotic, I don't know. Help clear some of the confusion away?'

Dr McCulloch hovered over her. 'Let's hold fire there a moment,' she said, shaking her head. 'Don't overdo it.'

'I'll record it as psychotic depression,' Afrah continued.

'Some other people have wondered about it before, so we're probably on to something.'

She stood up, her face drained of colour.

'I need a coffee break or I'm going to actually fall over. I'll be back in ten.'

I watched her disappear down the hallway. Dr McCulloch started humming.

'Will you see her too?' I asked her. 'I think some things were maybe . . . missed.'

She nodded knowingly. 'Afrah's been working non-stop for too long. I don't know if I'll have time though, unfortunately.' She looked genuinely pained.

How can this be right? I thought. *What is it we're doing if we don't have time to talk to the people who so desperately want to be heard? If we don't have time to decipher what they really need?*

'Could I talk to her then?'

Dr McCulloch tipped her head ruefully. 'Best not to be on your own here at this point,' she said. 'You're not covered by the insurance. It's a shame we've not got more time to offer her though. I might just have to give her a different medication.'

She seemed to read my disappointment.

'Oh, you should see how much worse it is with the private patients who float down here,' she told me. 'The private psychs put them on all sorts of medication which we have to try and wean them off, if we get a chance. Which, usually, we don't.'

'Really?' I said, surprised. I had wondered if private psychiatry, with fewer financial restrictions, might not rely so heavily on medication.

'Oh, *yes*.' She widened her eyes. 'You were under the illusion things are better in the private sector?' She nodded, as if to silence herself. 'Often quite the contrary.'

Later, I went up to the office to look for Afrah and spooked an agency nurse who'd been asleep on a chair.

'Shit!' he said, taking the jumper off his face.

He explained he'd just finished his night shift and asked where Afrah was. I noticed a half-eaten Twix bar in his hand.

'She's on a break,' I told him. 'I was just looking for her.'

He was silent as he finished the chocolate.

'Can you tell her I've seen eight people, and the other guy didn't turn up,' he said, using the Twix as a pointing device.

Eight assessments in one night, I thought. *That's a lot.*

The nurse crumpled the wrapper into his pocket. 'I'm already late finishing,' he said, wiping at the corners of his mouth.

While I waited for Afrah, I read through the nurse's assessments. It was bleak reading: multiple suicide attempts, panic attacks, domestic violence, sexual assault, abuse. A lot of devastation to hear, to record. Yet the recording itself was oddly threadbare, questions designed to be ticked through, perhaps to keep the staff as far removed from the pain as possible.

Maybe it wasn't meant to be an exercise in empathy and understanding; instead, we're encouraged to pick out *symptom*s, giving us as practitioners the ability to evade experiences that are too difficult to hear. Human distress can be flattened and erased this way, concentrating individual complexity into sterile boxes. This agency nurse's assessments sketched the contradiction at the heart of our job: we record and classify, but then what? And if this *is* the job, how do we do it sufficiently? Across several assessments, he'd replicated the same exact paragraph. On a few, he'd confused the Subjective impressions – information based on the practitioner's own opinion – and Objective impressions – the factual information. One whole new assessment had been copied and pasted word for word from another assessment the nurse had carried out two years before. These reports exemplified staff just going through the motions, getting through a shift like any other shift on any other job.

When Afrah returned, I showed her the assessments. She sighed deeply and was silent. I watched her sipping her coffee.

'Best to go mad in the daytime, if you can,' she said. 'Might have a better chance of getting decent treatment.'

It is routine for psychiatric liaison nurses, as we're known here, to be called from A&E to the general medicine wards. Often these calls come from the Burns Unit, where you must wear a head-to-toe plastic suit while asking intimate questions. Or it's a conversation through tangled tubes in the Intensive Care Unit after a suicide attempt, or the Maternity Unit, to see an inconsolable mother who's lost her baby. During these rounds I often noticed a curious lethargy to how general medical staff greeted us or considered our assessments. An incredulous glare, bordering just short of disdain. Mental health staff, it seemed, were thought to be at the bottom of the pile, their competence and doctrine quietly interrogated by the medics around them. In response, liaison nurses often equipped themselves with a prickly demeanour.

Despite the recurrent disregard for psychiatric staff, there were certain mental health diagnoses which could produce a palpable disquiet within general teams. On my fifth day in A&E I followed Dr McCulloch to a surgical ward. We'd been told that a man in his twenties had been admitted with severe stomach pain. That he was 'one of ours'.

We travelled up in a full lift, walked through the back door of the ward and curved past a man in scrubs pushing an empty bed. Across the hallway, a chiselled young doctor was standing next to a filing cabinet holding a clipboard. He walked skittishly towards us.

'Thanks for coming so quickly.' He breathed out when he reached us, sounding genuinely relieved.

Dr McCulloch nodded. 'Of course. Schizophrenia?' she replied, nonchalantly.

The doctor seemed to stiffen. 'Well,' he said, sounding out the vowel. 'He seemed *normal* at first, but when we checked his records, we saw the diagnosis.' He paused, slowing himself. 'I'm not sure how unwell he is, but there were mentions of ... *violence*. And he went AWOL from an Acute Ward about three months ago, it appears. He was being given a regular depot injection, zuclopenthixol 500mg, but he's long overdue now. I wasn't sure what to do.'

Dr McCulloch continued to nod, letting a silence expand between them. I wondered if a part of her enjoyed the doctor's nervous attentiveness.

'Hmm,' she said, 'AWOL?'

'Erm, yes,' the doctor replied. 'I asked him about it, whether he'd taken any medication in the last three months, and he said he'd had horrible side effects. He ... well, he actually *begged* me not to make him take it.'

Dr McCulloch made a drawn-out noise. The young doctor was flicking the corner of his clipboard repetitively. I saw her notice this, her eyes squinting.

'OK, and what about oral medication?' she asked.

'Not taking any, apparently. But he said he'd take oral olanzapine if he must. He just doesn't want his depot again.'

'Got it. Any CTO?'

Community Treatment Order – another term I recognized from my introductory weeks. A patient diagnosed with a mental disorder can be forced by law to abide by their clinician's treatment plan when outside hospital, regardless of whether they agree with their diagnosis or consent to taking the medication prescribed, which is usually in the form of a long-acting antipsychotic depot injection.

'No.' The young doctor shook his head. 'Not that we could find in his records.'

'Right.' Dr McCulloch looked thoughtful. 'Was he aggressive in any way?'

'Not really, no. He was very agitated, but he's in a lot of pain, so that's not unusual. We wanted to sedate him due to the pain but wondered if you should assess him first.'

The doctor passed her the clipboard containing the patient information. There were dark stains beneath his armpits.

'Not a problem,' Dr McCulloch said. 'Good that you called us.'

'Oh,' said the doctor. 'Of course, thank you for your swiftness.'

There was a brief silence as Dr McCulloch glanced over the top sheet of paper. 'I'll go through all this and then pop right over,' she replied. 'Don't sedate him yet.'

The doctor shook his head. 'No, no, definitely. We won't.'

*

THE HALLWAY

The skinny, wide-eyed man behind the curtain was curled up on the bed, clutching his stomach. He moaned when we asked his name.

'I'm sorry, Javon,' Dr McCulloch said, moving closer. 'Horrible to be in so much pain.'

Javon nodded, his face contorted.

'We're going to ask some questions,' she continued. 'Just to see how you're doing and find out what you need, OK? Nothing you haven't been asked many times before, I'm sure. But we just want to see how best to help you.'

The man looked at us and I noticed the whites of his eyes were slightly yellowed. His matching tracksuit, too, looked like a faded hue of its previous shade.

'*Please*, doctor,' he said, 'I just want this to stop. *Please*.'

Dr McCulloch carried out a full mental assessment and found Javon to have capacity. If you are regarded as lacking capacity because of a mental disturbance, decisions about your care will be made for you. Yet Javon was found to legally have the ability to weigh up information and make evaluations, and he showed no signs of delusion, psychosis or risk to himself or others. The doctor concluded that he was dishevelled, undernourished and without a fixed abode, but despite not being on any psychiatric medication for months he was in fact currently mentally well. She communicated this to the young doctor, tension visibly evacuating his angular frame.

Javon was sedated, and the surgery scheduled.

Dr McCulloch finished her shift. The doctor finished his shift. I finished my shift.

*

When I returned the next morning, I found Afrah in the office sipping black coffee from a cup shaped like a cartoon M&M. Her hair looked unbrushed, and there was heavy concealer around her eyes. She raised her hand lethargically when she saw me and I sat down opposite her.

'You're still here?' I asked, concerned.

Afrah nodded and put her cup down. 'You know,' she said, not looking at me, 'I can't say this anywhere official, but doesn't mean it isn't true.' She bit the side of her lip and continued to look ahead. 'So, that kid, Javon. The medical team that took over last night – they read about his diagnosis, his medical history. They saw that dreaded word written down – *schizophrenia*. I think they panicked.' She looked at me for the first time. '*I* think that all-white team saw his brown face and his diagnosis and they freaked out. They operated, and even though the notes said he should've got a stoma due to risk of organ failure and infection, they didn't give him one. No, they said, they were worried a man with *schizophrenia* would mess with it, pull it out.'

I heard myself inhale sharply. '*No.*'

'Oh, it gets worse.' Afrah shook her head. 'Then, while he's still asleep, they just go ahead and inject that boy with 500mg of zuclopenthixol. They didn't even use the 100mg safety restart dose.'

'No,' I said again, stunned.

'So, I asked them after, "What happened?" They just said they were worried he would go crazy on them.'

I thought back to the evening before, how small and helpless Javon had seemed lying curled on that bed.

'Will there be any disciplinary action?' I asked.

Afrah shook her head. 'No,' she said, slowly. 'Nothing will happen. It's too . . . messy.'

In certain phases of sleep, our mind processes the day through abstract dream play. While we exist between the conscious and unconscious, we form meaning and comprehension from chaos. We assemble and compile our experiences so they become memories, the building blocks to understanding ourselves and the world. But it is in sleep that we are also most vulnerable.

This waking nightmare belongs to Javon. But the truth of his experience exists within a frightening hall of mirrors. With so many involved, we struggle to tease out culpability: there is no easy finger to point. If a diagnosis carries with it the threat of danger, the person obscured by it can be rendered voiceless. If information exchange is multiple or unclear, we can invent our own script. When a person can be othered, it's easier not to treat them as we would ourselves.

'Nothing will happen,' Afrah said again. 'Bits have been reported, but no one will take it any further. I wish I could tell you otherwise.'

It was close to midnight the next evening when three first-year art students arrived in A&E. They huddled silently in a corner of the room, avoiding eye contact. A boy in dungarees signed in Daisy, a striking young woman with pink hair, before shuffling back into the cluster.

'She's smoked a lot of spice by accident,' the boy said to a doctor's chest. 'Something's happened to her.'

A&E is busiest after dark. There is something about the closing of a day which brings panic, the receding of hope. But

Daisy was dancing with joy, her ringed fingers reaching up to the ceiling, her rainbow skirt twisting around her.

'My heart is pumping!' she exclaimed in a clipped accent. '*Boom, boom, boom!*'

Afrah had gone home, and the nurse I was with watched Daisy as she bent down and started wiping the floor rhythmically. Laughing and then, suddenly, crying.

'There they are!' Daisy proclaimed, a tear dripping on to the back of her hand. She stared into the floor for a moment, and then laughed again. 'Look! They're not from this world!' She turned to us, beaming. Her face wet. 'Amazing!' she said, shaking her head, before resuming her wiping.

The nurse turned to me. 'Looks like a simple one,' she said. 'Bipolar, first presentation – I feel it in my gut.'

I looked back at Daisy. She was singing.

'Hasn't she just smoked a load of spice?' I asked, perplexed by the nurse's confidence.

The nurse nodded. 'The drugs can bring on an underlying mania. Happens all the time.'

There was a tautness to her words, a noticeable impatience.

'She's just the *type* as well,' she continued. 'You have to look for the other signs.'

The nurse pulled a pad and pen from her back pocket.

'Can you go and get the psychiatrist on duty to come down?' she said. 'I'm gonna start with her.'

When I finally located the psychiatrist, a woman I'd not met wearing high-heeled shoes and a pencil skirt, twenty minutes had passed. We went down to the ward and found Daisy doing yogic stretches, talking to herself. The nurse put her hands up in mock despair and walked towards us. The psychiatrist looked over at Daisy, and then read through the nurse's assessment. I read over her shoulder.

Inappropriately dressed, the nurse had written. *Wearing a skirt over trousers and lots of necklaces. Some evidence of self-neglect.*

'What evidence of self-neglect?' I asked.

The nurse looked at me and then quickly away. 'You should be *noticing* these things as a nurse,' she remarked.

I watched Daisy taking off her shoes, then her socks, before cradling her bare feet.

'I think you might have to give me a hint.'

The nurse made a clucking sound. 'Her hands are *dirty*. Her nails are *dirty*. Her skirt is *dirty*.'

I looked back at Daisy. She looked like any other regular art student.

The psychiatrist folded the assessment and slid it under her clipboard. 'OK,' she said. 'I'll see her now.'

The nurse had got the number for Daisy's mum from the shuffling friends, and we called her at home from the reception. The woman on the end of the line sounded panicked, her voice thin and reedy. 'There's no history of mental health issues in the family!' she told us. She didn't know her daughter took drugs. 'We'll be *right there*,' she said. '*Please*, use our private medical insurance if she needs anything. Put her in a private bed until she calms down, until she sleeps it off.'

The nurse put the phone down as the psychiatrist approached us.

'She's totally psychotic,' the psychiatrist informed us, and yawned. 'She started telling me she's recording an album. Thinks she's a famous singer.'

On a hunch, I used my phone to look Daisy up online. YouTube videos popped up, a Bandcamp site.

'She *is* releasing an album,' I told the psychiatrist. 'She's a folk singer.'

'Oh, well, regardless,' she continued, waving a hand dismissively. 'She's manic. She needs to go to an Acute Ward.'

I was stunned. *How often are diagnoses constructed from unchecked assumptions?*

The nurse made a noise in agreement. 'The mum sounded like a rich snob,' she said to the psychiatrist. 'I don't know if she's telling the truth about the family history. Probably doesn't want the *stigma*.'

The psychiatrist raised an eyebrow. 'Good, well. Let's find her a bed somewhere.'

Three hours later, no bed had been found, and Daisy's family had arrived. A clustering of mother, father, sister around the bed Daisy was sat cross-legged on, drawing pictures in red pen and singing to herself.

'She just needs to come home for a bit.' Her mum was shaking as she pulled the curtain across. 'She doesn't need a *mental hospital*. She's not *ill*.'

They refused the sedative the psychiatrist advised.

The nurse told them about bipolar disorder, explained that an antipsychotic would help her come down from the mania, as the sister cried quietly into the hospital blanket.

No, they said. *We'll wait it out. That's all she needs.*

More hours passed, and no acute bed could be located. I found myself hoping the hours would tick by without success, realizing with a jolt that a part of me wanted Daisy to run from us, to get away as quickly as possible. *But aren't we helping people?* I thought. *Aren't we keeping them, and others, safe?*

It was late morning the next day when Daisy finally fell asleep, her sister curled at her feet. Her parents were raw-eyed, their jaws tense with exhaustion, when Dr McCulloch started her shift.

When Daisy woke up, her face smeared with ink, she assessed her. Daisy was quiet now, her arms around her sister whose hair was stuck to one side of her face with tears and sleep. Forty minutes later, discharge papers were signed. There was a tentative recommendation to speak to the Home Treatment Team, and a prescription for the sedative zopiclone to help her sleep again.

'You had the doctor-in-charge last night *very* concerned,' Dr McCulloch told them. She turned towards me. 'She's all right. They can go.'

The nurse from last night was standing next to me. I could feel the anger radiating from her as she sneered at the doctor's back. 'That girl will be back,' she said under her breath. 'What a mistake.'

I moved away from her, ignoring her mutterings behind me.

Dr McCulloch sat down behind the reception area and unfolded the glasses that hung around her neck. I sat next to her, a palpable relief moving through me.

'I'm so glad you're here,' I whispered, feeling a sudden desire to cling to her.

Dr McCulloch looked at me. 'Tough night?' she said, her forehead knotting.

'I mean, how can anyone be assessed for a mental illness while on drugs? It seems crazy.'

'Well,' she sighed, 'it depends on the practitioner really. On what stance they take as to whether a person has an underlying condition that's been *activated* by the drug, or if it's just the drug.'

'But, how can you tell that?'

'Hmm,' she said, looking weary. 'Clinical judgement? Personal beliefs?'

I was fizzing with incredulity, unable to let it pass. 'So, this could have gone either way?' I persisted. 'Her parents refused the medication, and they couldn't find a bed, which meant her sleeping here and you seeing her, and—'

'Yes,' she interrupted. 'Often the case.'

*

In psychiatry, the rapid categorizing of someone's distress into a diagnosis is usually crucial. The first time you meet a person in A&E you're asked to codify their 'illness' via a series of box ticks. Diagnosis, of course, exists across medicine to enable quick treatment. However, mental health is different. There are no physical tests for diagnosis, only the judgement of a mental health practitioner with all our moral values, prejudices, potential lack of skill or adequate training, and exhaustion levels. Yet despite this, as nurses and psychiatrists we are not taught to adequately question these biases in ourselves. Instead, we're trained to see ourselves as the expert, and the person in front of us as lacking capacity to understand themselves, or what's best for them.

A psychiatric diagnosis, though sometimes embraced, can also produce a profound loss of personal meaning. The label can obscure or sever us from the experiences and stories which shine a light on *why* we are emotionally distressed, and in turn restrict our agency to alter anything. A diagnosis can also have an insidious effect on how practitioners engage with a person. Grouping someone into a category impacts on whether their opinion is or isn't believed, what treatment is and isn't available, how dangerous they are deemed, whether they are sectioned against their will, which medication, what doses, and whether it is offered, coerced or forced. A diagnosis can remove a person's reliability, and once recorded in their file the assertion is like a worm, burrowing into all future judgements and decisions.

*

Afrah moved more sanguinely that morning, a little swing in her arms which had previously seemed weighed down. She'd changed into another flannel shirt, and there was a steaming cup of coffee in her hand.

'Sleep,' she cooed, 'wonderful sleep.'

I told her about the evening before.

'Interesting,' she said. 'And not unusual. Last week a man came in with ketamine-induced psychosis and the locum psychiatrist diagnosed him with schizophrenia on the second day. He put him on olanzapine. Then it's kind of difficult to know if he calmed down because of the antipsychotic or if the ketamine just wore off.'

A flush of anger gripped me. 'Daisy's family seemed to stop

a lot of those things happening – the drugs, the treatment teams...'

Afrah studied me. 'Yeah.' She paused. 'If the person's been picked up on their own, if no one else can tell you anything – no family or whatever – and they're out of their mind at this point, then practitioners will just make a call. It's much better when they're brought in by ambulance. They're more likely to get a piss and blood test to eliminate drugs and other organic reasons for their behaviour. You'd *think* this was always checked, but it's not. At least, not that I've always seen.'

A security guard was standing opposite us, his hand on his radio. 'Someone needs to see this girl pretty soon,' he said to us, sounding irritated. 'She's going into every single cubicle, and tried to get into ICU when I turned my back.'

*

I didn't want to write about this admission. I so badly want it not to have happened, not to have been someone's reality. I almost walked away from the course that evening, when the shreds of meaning I'd been clinging to fell away. *What was I doing here?* I felt like a blundering tourist in an immutable ecosystem; I sensed the absurdity of my footfall, my deluded participation. *What was I looking for?* Do we seek out encounters with difference to encounter ourselves differently? Had I wanted to stand right up close to the shapeless complexity of the human condition to enable my own outline to be drawn more clearly? I feel so guilty that I was able to walk away, though the memory still hugs me like skin. I try to console myself by believing I did something consequential, but I'm filled with rage at how close we came to colluding. At how this story I'm trying so hard to quell with words represents thousands of stories like it, none of them fixed on the page, their outcomes unknown.

*

Uma wouldn't sit down. She was pacing the hallway, businesslike. Opening and closing curtains as if she expected something or someone to surprise her there. She was slender and in her early twenties, wearing the neat, professional clothes of an office worker. Her make-up was precise, her hair fastened. Her boss had brought her into A&E minutes earlier. I'd seen his twisted, anxious face as he walked away from the central reception. Uma hadn't said goodbye. She was busy pacing, inspecting, mumbling to herself.

Afrah was called away, and I didn't check with anyone first, as I normally would, before approaching her. I felt emboldened by what had happened with Daisy, my anger – as Alex said it would – fuelling me. A general distrust, it seemed, had been gnawing at me. I watched Uma moving, muttering, and felt a sharp pang of protectiveness. I called her name. She looked up at me with a calm absence, without any simulation of the rules of engagement.

'Wait. Wait. Wait,' she said instead, without intonation.

I stopped walking. 'You'd like me to wait?' I asked.

'W-ay-ta. W-ay-ta.' She sounded out the parts this time, as if she'd liked how they'd felt in her mouth. Then she walked past me.

A nurse came over, her arms outstretched as if she was

corralling sheep. 'Sorry!' she called. 'You need to go into this room, please!'

The nurse pulled back a curtain and waved Uma out of the hallway and into the cubicle. Uma followed purposefully, as the nurse turned back towards reception, leaving us together. I watched Uma moving around the cubicle, inspecting each corner of the bed, fingering the folds in the sheet. She picked up the pillow and put it down again.

'No. No. No,' she murmured, circling the bed.

I watched her, curious. Her presentation – smart white shirt, gold necklace, spotless black pumps – seemed so at odds with her absence of social affectation, like a child entirely within her own world. Unplugged, offline.

I tried to ask Uma if she knew where she was. Where she'd been that morning. She answered with thoughtful non sequiturs.

The nurse appeared at the curtain line again, frowning. 'The locum consultant will be here in a few minutes,' she said. 'Afrah's asked if you'd help her with the man in cubicle four.'

I nodded, not wanting to leave, trying to remember which curtained area that was. I turned back to Uma. She had pushed her trousers down to her ankles and was bent back over the bed. Her hips thrust into the air.

'Uma!' I said, moving quickly towards her. 'Let's put these back on.'

A pulse of alarm moved through me. *Why was she undressing?*

As I helped Uma pull up her trousers, I noticed a yellowing bruise splayed across her hip. I asked her what happened.

For a second, she looked at me. Something connected. Some light turned on.

'*Stop*,' she whispered.

'OK!' A locum consultant was standing in front of us. 'Hello, erm, Uma.' He peered over his glasses as she stood up and began circling the bed again. 'Thanks,' he said to me politely. 'I'm just going to have a rudimentary chat before we call any next of kin. You can leave us.'

I left Uma with the consultant reluctantly, and couldn't concentrate in cubicle four, where Afrah was conducting a capacity assessment on an old man found wandering in a shopping centre. I kept seeing Uma's eyes in that moment, how they'd seemed to be pleading, reaching beyond words. What was happening in there? What story would that doctor narrate for this young, inaudible girl? How was I already so distrustful of our capabilities, of the sturdiness of our tenet?

Uma's boss had left the only contact he had been given: 'Daddy'.

Afrah and I were in the reception area when the consultant called him. He spoke kindly, informing him that Uma was here and safe. That he was yet to conduct a full assessment, but that on initial inspection she was very unwell and would likely need to go to a mental health hospital to be treated for psychosis. Daddy sounded calm. He thanked the consultant for his expertise, praising his advice. Then he asked firmly that the doctor not speak to Uma any more, to wait until he got there. 'I don't want to *miss* anything,' I heard him say. 'I want to be there to *support* her.'

The consultant put down the phone and smiled. 'OK, good,' he said. 'The father is on his way to help. The girl's barely vocal at the moment, sadly, so it will be very useful to have him here. Let's wait a bit to assess her. The poor man sounds stiff with worry.'

I knew I was meant to wait for Daddy to come. But something made me uneasy, like the metronomic tick of a bomb. Perhaps it was what happened to Daisy – what almost happened. So I didn't wait. I went straight back into the cubicle. There, I found Uma lying on the floor on her back, her legs bunched up under her, her arms above her head. I've blurred this memory almost beyond comprehension. It exists now in a series of stills, of five-second film, distress having drugged its reality from me. It still resurfaces sometimes, now, years later, in flashes of movement, in bruised flesh around wrists, ankles. Red-hot rope burns, hidden under fabric.

What happened? I kept asking. *What happened?*

Uma was crying now. *Daddy*, she kept repeating. *Can't get away.*

'Your dad?' I asked, nausea rising. 'Your dad can't get away?'

'Make him *stop*. Make him *stop*.'

'Stop?'

She looked at me again, her eyes boring into me. '*Can't get* . . .' she growled, '*away* . . .'

Uma started to take her trousers down again, started to mime, to thrust. Pinning her bruised wrists together above her head. Tears streaming down her cheeks.

Help me, she whispered.

I remember running down the hallway. Breathless, dizzy. Telling Afrah, telling the consultant to stop him. To not let Daddy in. To protect her. The bruises, the rope burns. *Stop him.*

The next half an hour remains a haze of panic and

movement. Of phone calls and inspections and questions. The horrified look on Afrah's face. The consultant shaking his head, checking his notes repeatedly, as if he'd find something there that would make this all go away.

Security are alerted. The police are called. Everything moves fast. Slow. Fast. Unreal. Daddy is stopped at the entrance. He fights, thrashing out. He tries to run.

Afrah was watching me. I'd been sitting in the office for over an hour, unable to do anything at all except stare at the wall.

'I think,' she said to me, her forehead creasing, 'you need to get out of here for a while.'

I looked up at her.

'No, *really*,' she said. 'You need a break.' She put her hand on my shoulder.

I swallowed. Unable to say anything and keep myself together.

'You're going back to the Acute Ward next week, right? Maybe just take the rest of today off, it's your last day anyway. Just slip out.' She nodded. 'Honestly. Take some time away from all this.'

*

That weekend is a blank, my life on hold. Sleeping and waking blurs; broken, disturbed. I can only remember the sharp smell of the Acute Ward's reception again on the Monday morning. The muted recognition of the security guard at the door. My footsteps in the hallway. With unexpected, unsettling relief, I was back.

Yet in my head I was with Uma. Playing and replaying those moments. Wishing they were different, fighting images as they leapt at me, the recollections bringing a confused kind of terror, as if I were isolated beneath a bell jar from the world.

I know how possible it is that the notes about Daddy were pushed to the back of Uma's story while practitioners on whatever ward she was sectioned busied themselves treating her 'psychotic illness'. They could so easily be buried under new observations, assumed to be insignificant with the passing of time.

Memories of trauma are so fragile, if someone told me this experience didn't happen, I would question myself immediately. If someone told me again and again that it didn't happen, if they told me I'd been *unwell* at that time, that I'd imagined it, I would probably believe them. So much of me would be grateful to relinquish its truth, rather than revive it. But I am the fortunate one, the one with the power. Uma will be burdened by her trauma for a lifetime. I only have to live with knowing I didn't follow up after this moment. I didn't search for her. I didn't call around wards and consultants, making sure again and again that she was safe, that her story was believed. I just walked away. But she didn't let me go. She still hasn't let me go.

*

Back on the ward, I walked down the familiar hallway into the day area in a fog. A wiry man with one arm and one leg in plaster was sitting at an empty table, his crutches resting

THE HALLWAY

against his good leg. Two other men, one on each sofa, were slumped in silence, their eyes fixed on the flashing TV screen. The images of suntanned bodies and smiling, beautiful faces like some cruel dream. Beside them, a nurse perched on one arm of the sofa, her finger scanning across her phone. I watched them, dazed.

A loud slam broke my spell, a door colliding with a wall. Everyone in the room turned.

'Come on!' someone yelled. 'I'm ready for you!'

The man was dressed in camouflage. He wore sunglasses, a green woollen hat, leather gloves and a camo backpack. His neck and half of his face – the only visible parts of his body – were almost translucent in their pallor. Some tufts of hair, a dusty shade of orange, tangled out below the thick wool.

'Watch out!' he screamed into the empty hallway. 'I can blast through any shield!'

His frame was approaching the day area, stiff limbs marching. An invisible automatic weapon in his gloved hands.

'Just watch me, I'm the Emancipator!' he barked like a preacher addressing a congregation.

I watched him moving towards me, transfixed. The unreality of the scene numbing my senses like a decompression chamber. *I'm back*, I thought.

Noticing me, the man stopped just a few metres away. I couldn't see his eyes through the sheen of his dark lenses, but I knew he was surveying me. Another nurse appeared from a doorway, turned and disappeared again.

He was walking towards me. I froze.

'Oh, *hello*,' he said calmly, sticking out a hand for me to shake and pushing his sunglasses on to his forehead. 'I'm Rich.'

I hesitated, trying to compute his sudden change in demeanour.

'It's nice to meet you,' he said. 'You're a student?'

I nodded, my chest rising and falling.

He paused and scanned my face, searching for something. 'One . . . second . . .' He held up a leather finger.

I watched his eyes narrow as he looked up and down the hallway. Seeing no one, he turned to me again.

'That's . . . nice to hear. *Very* nice actually,' he said.

There was a pause as we studied each other. I tried to guess his age, but he was ageless. There was something innocent yet cadaverous about him.

Then his arm shot out and he grasped mine tightly. The breath caught in my throat as I tried to speak.

'Please,' he whispered, urgently, pulling me a few feet further away from the office. '*Please*. Don't listen to the staff here. Don't see us as a diagnosis. Ask *us* who we are, what *we* think . . . we're the ones with the problem, we know more than them.'

Rich's focus shifted to somewhere over my head. I turned to see Fuad, who smiled at us as he walked past.

'Welcome back,' he said to me.

'All right, Fuad?' Rich replied, giving him a queen's wave.

Fuad twirled his hand in a mock regal gesture.

There was a pause as he disappeared into a room.

'That's a good man there,' Rich said. 'But there are some devils working in mental health.' He shook his head slowly. 'I've been in the system for twenty years. I've had kidney failure, seizures from all the drugs they've given me. I'm barely alive.'

THE HALLWAY

An agency nurse appeared across the hall and called to me. Rich watched as I smiled at her, told her I'd be right there. When I looked back at him, his face had fallen.

'You . . . you won't ever forget what I'm saying to you, will you?' He seemed fragile, suddenly, despite his imposing physique. 'Don't let them make you forget.'

For much of the following week, Rich paced the hallways shouting intimidations at alien invaders. Red patches of anger rising up his neck, his breathing shallow, his voice rasping. At times the weapon in his empty hands had a shotgun action, at others it was a rapid-fire machine gun. Isolated and under siege, he would be impenetrable, sensing a threat so pervasive that to him it was otherworldly.

Yet, one afternoon, he was utterly beaten.

After crying for hours in the hallway, he asked to speak to me, alone.

Rich had asked to open 'The Chill-Out' – one of two vacant, locked rooms either side of the day area – and dragged another chair in for me. I watched him through the glass, unmoving, his head in his hands. His gloves and sunglasses on the floor beside him.

I knew I wasn't meant to be on my own with a patient unless in the hallway, and felt a wave of unexpected fear, followed by a tug of shame at this admission. I looked around, seeking some kind of reassurance, and saw Ray coming out of the day area. I caught her before she slipped back into the office.

'Is it OK for me to talk to Rich in there?'

She looked at me, tilting her head with an air of curiosity.

'Yes, OK. Just keep the door slightly open and sit close to it. See what he wants – it's good he wants to speak about it, whatever it is. And if you feel unsafe in any way, just pull your alarm.'

I had forgotten about the heavy plastic pendulum hanging around my neck. I hadn't liked wearing it from the start – it seemed too much on display, like an emblem of pessimism, a label declaring my distrust of the people around me.

I clasped the smooth alarm in my palm and walked towards the room.

'Rich?'

I opened the door and he looked up from his hands. His face red and blotched.

'Can I tell you something?' he said, his tone pleading, the palms of his hands pressed together in his lap.

I stepped in, my whole body tense. 'Of course.'

Rich said he wanted to die. He told me he had no qualifications, having been diagnosed with depression as a teenager and then swiftly sectioned to a ward and given his first antipsychotic medication. He explained he wasn't able to do his exams because of the heavy sedation the drugs caused, and now in his early forties he had no hope for a future. He'd been in and out of hospital all his life, never seeming to get well, and had now been sectioned for five months with a renewal hanging over him.

'I don't know why I'm thinking about the past now,' he said to the floor between us. 'I had a dream last night about first going into hospital. I didn't feel ... I didn't feel like anyone wanted me, does that make sense? I felt like everyone must've hated me, that I was completely useless. That I needed to be silenced.'

THE HALLWAY

The ward was still around us.

'What were they silencing?'

Rich rocked his head back. 'Oh, I don't know . . . just *me*. My thoughts. My life. And things were pretty terrible at home, you know.' He paused. 'Then the government started turning me into a cyborg year by year. They pumped me full of secret fuel, now I'm mostly machine.'

I watched him chew at the inside of his cheek.

'What medication did they put you on?'

He clenched his fists. 'Oh, they have me full of everything. Haloperidol, quetiapine, clonazepam, lorazepam, sertraline, procyclidine.'

I checked these through in my head: two antipsychotics, two benzodiazepines, an antidepressant and a medication to reduce the side effects of the others.

'Now I need meds for life,' he continued. 'I can't sleep without them. I can't be me without them. I've been on them too long, they've changed the chemicals in my brain. I don't know who I am without drugs any more.'

I nodded, a knot of sadness in my throat.

'Besides, I need it to be *activated* for duty.'

Rich explained he'd been given a secret mission he defined as 'saving the world', an onerous task which filled him with pride and significance. It was as if his portentous delusions were a coping mechanism for dealing with the loneliness and futility which plagued him. His body's reliance on medication, and the story he'd told himself about its force and necessity, confirming his inhuman form.

'You must have complex feelings about psychiatry,' I managed, feeling helpless.

He nodded emphatically. 'Well, the system is part of the government. You see, they're surveying me ... injecting me. I'm one of their *projects*.'

His eyes drifted away, and I noticed his arms, like most of the patients', were shaking. A common antipsychotic drug side effect. He clasped them protectively, and took a long breath in.

'But I'm deployed for life. I can't go off duty now, or they'll hang me.'

We sat together in silence. It felt palpable, suffocating.

'I'm so sorry,' I said, finally.

Rich started to cry. 'It's never gonna change,' he whispered. 'Because, because – the nurses are so cold. Most of them just come and do their shifts. There are a few angels, some who actually care and worry and listen. But the others, why don't they go and work in Asda if it's just a job for them?'

My head felt like a helium balloon as I grasped around for something to say, straining to stay with him in his devastation. A rush of jumbled sentences came and went. I wanted to tell him it would be OK, I wanted to say things would get better; but I knew the words were meaningless. I knew they would benefit me more than him. My body tense and exhausted, I felt wretched. Useless.

'Thank you for listening to me,' he said, his eyes finding mine for the first time.

I swallowed. 'Of course,' I said. 'Any time you want to speak...'

He smiled weakly and stood up, before leaving me in the empty room.

*

Some days later, Rich was back marching along the hallway again. He saw me and stopped a few feet away, looked over my shoulder, ducked, and pulled the trigger of an invisible pistol several times.

'Got them!' he exclaimed, smiling.

Without thinking I saluted him, and he laughed. A loud, guttural laugh that reverberated off the stark walls.

I felt my face flush. 'Sorry,' I said. 'That just felt right somehow.'

'Yeah,' he said, grinning, 'it was.'

I asked how he was feeling.

'Back on task with an important job to do!'

He rubbed his hands together vigorously, forgetting his gun. I noticed his eyes were unfocused, his pale hands still trembling.

He paused.

'But this place . . .' Rich looked around the hallway suspiciously, then through the doorway of the day area. The man with crutches was sat alone at his regular table, sipping coffee from a blue plastic cup. Three others were slumped on the sofas. Rich lowered his voice. 'I want to get out now *so* badly, but I don't want to go to assisted living. It's so, *so* horrible. It's frightening, dirty, full of scary people – seriously. People get beaten up there, touched up, raped there . . . and it's supposed to be a place that supports you.'

He looked back at the sofa people in silence. I watched his hand shaking at his side.

'These people. I've spent so many years looking into the eyes of people like these, every day, seeing their pain. It's torture.'

Behind Rich, Dr Oxley, trailed by two trainee psychiatrists, was moving along the hallway towards us. They passed silently into the day area, stopping to stand in the far corner. We watched the doctor gesticulate, his voice muffled by the television, and point at the patient sat alone in the corner. The students nodded keenly.

'New students,' Rich whispered, shaking his head. 'To be educated in the way of the doctor. It just goes on and on . . .'

4

The Bedroom

For most of us, a bedroom is the first place we can call our own. There, we begin to comprehend ourselves as separate, unique – it is a canvas for invention. I remember how, as a child, curation within those walls became my way to exist; I could reflect my burgeoning internal world back to myself, to others. This poster, this scrawled quote, this book, this colour – this is *me*.

We can construct reality within those walls, we can hide. We can escape to safety from a tumultuous home – our first comprehension of the wider world.

I struggle to recall the bedrooms on the Acute Ward; the uniformity has erased them from my mind. Some contained multiple beds behind white curtains; most held a single bed, a bedside table, nothing more. I avoided them. Perhaps because they remained echoes of possibility, never fulfilled. But they were also places of fear, of danger – for staff, for patients. As if physical space could absorb a person's trauma and distress, and venturing inside would overpower us.

*

'Seriously, I've had enough of her,' the nurse said, sitting down across from me in the office.

Ray nodded in response, as an agency nurse shuffled in and positioned herself by the radiator.

Two others murmured in agreement.

'She's rude and demanding,' one of them added.

'That's personality disorder for you,' offered the other.

Alice was a woman in her sixties with the top-heavy body of an Olympic swimmer, a frizz of red hair and an elegant public-schooled voice. She had been pulled off the streets by police officers after she'd refused to go with them to a shelter.

Alice claimed she slept rough by choice, professing to own two uninhabited houses which she declined to live in. The confusion this admission caused to everyone she spoke to preceded a wave of disbelief and concern, followed by grating irritation. She was, they felt, delusional if she *didn't* own two houses, and delusional if she *did* but insisted on 'acting' homeless. Her rejection of the police officer's desire to rescue her – a vulnerable older woman – from the streets disconcerted him enough to deploy Section 136, the mandate allowing officers to hold a person by force if they suspect them of having a mental disorder.

Alice had arrived in the middle of the night, fiercely indignant. She screamed that she'd been wronged. That it was immoral. 'You *bastards* don't have any right to force me,' she sneered. 'I demand to be released immediately.'

Though, by the third day, Alice appeared as if on holiday. She trimmed and painted her toenails, ate two portions of dessert and read the newspaper in her pyjamas. She refused to speak to staff she disliked, and treated staff she approved of like colleagues, recommending they take notice of something another patient could benefit from, or pointing out tasks they should have done. She told us she'd worked in social care in the past, that she *understood hardship*.

'I mean,' the nurse continued to Ray, 'she was telling me you hadn't taken a patient out for leave yesterday. Seriously, that woman is a shit-stirrer.'

A short while later I found Alice sat on a chair in her bedroom reading the paper, her shoeless feet resting on the adjacent bed, a coffee beside her. I watched as she dipped her finger into the cup and sucked the warm liquid from the end of it. She looked up at me.

'Morning,' she called across the room, waving.

I returned the greeting and walked in through the open door, asking if I could sit down. She pulled at another chair near by without shifting her position. I asked how she was.

'Well!' she began cheerfully. 'I'm still waiting to be told I can *leave*. I'm still waiting to be told my cousin isn't trying to steal my house. I'm still writing letters to the lawyers, who are still ignoring me ... so, busy, really.' She smiled and tapped the handbag on the floor beside her. Wads of paper spilt from the open zip.

Alice told me she'd been writing letters to lawyers for years, trying to bring a case against her cousin, who she said was using her houses without her permission and refusing to give her any rent. According to other staff, her papers were shambolic and incoherent, and she'd never got anywhere with the case. They called this a *delusion* used to bolster her *grand opinion* of herself. In all likelihood, I'd been told repeatedly, she didn't even own these houses.

Alice, however, was adamant.

'But,' she continued, 'I should be having a meeting with a consultant today, and then we'll get to the bottom of all this.' She sipped her coffee.

I felt a sadness move through me: her optimism highlighted its paucity within these walls.

'Where will you go when you're discharged?' I asked, trying to mirror her sentiment.

She looked at me, perplexed. 'Go? Back to my spot, of course.' She pushed at her frizz of hair with the palm of her hand. 'My friends have been looking after my things for me.'

Alice had described her 'spot' to me the day before, explaining how the police had ruined the delicate shelter she'd built there. 'It was *painstaking*,' she'd said. '*Weeks* of work.'

'Do you mean, by the coffee shop?' I asked, hoping she would tell me about somewhere else. I couldn't think of her sleeping out in the open without accompanying violent images of what could happen to her.

'Yes,' she nodded happily. 'My alfresco bedroom. I miss it.'

I looked at her with her socks and coffee and paper.

She tilted her head. 'You're surprised,' she said fixedly. 'Sounds strange to you, right?'

'It's that . . .' I tried carefully. 'I mean, don't you get cold? Or, scared out there?'

Alice laughed, her head rocking backwards. Her mouth shining with silver fillings. 'No, silly! I have a lot of blankets, really good ones that friends gifted to me. I'm not scared, I'm never alone, there are always people around, people to talk to.' She pointed at the cup as if it was evidence. 'People buy me coffees and sit with me. They invite me to their homes. It's such a lovely area and people there have really smart homes. There're always people about, people to *worry* about me.'

This sounded so reasonable that for a moment I forgot that the bedroom she'd described was made of cardboard and wood and bits of old car.

'But, what about . . . your houses?' I asked, not for the first time.

'Look,' She uncrossed her legs and repositioned herself. 'What's the alternative? I live in a big old house all on my own? Which I've done before. No one comes to visit, no one cares. I get miserable, I see no one. I have no close family. What's the good in that? Sleeping out in the open is good for me. I'm . . . part of somewhere . . . part of something.' She opened her arms wide. 'But these miserable bastards here. These wretched nurses and doctors. They think their life makes more sense than mine? Pah. That's a *hoot*. Who's mad now? The one in the miserable job, miserable home, miserable relationship, convincing themselves that they're happy, or me?'

From somewhere outside the room I heard Alex's familiar voice. 'Saul,' he was saying, 'I got this for you.' I felt an excitement bubble through me. So much had happened since I'd last seen Alex, and I felt desperate to share it.

I excused myself and left Alice's bedroom. Saul and Alex were standing in the hallway and I waved as I sped up towards them.

'Mate,' Saul was saying, 'twenty-three hours and *done*.'

When I reached them, both Alex and Saul were grinning.

'You're back!' I said to Alex, elated.

He nodded. 'Yup. For a week.'

Saul tucked a small pad of paper into his pocket. 'Thanks buddy.' He looked from Alex to me. 'I'm gonna write a bucket list now shit is finally happenin' for me.'

'What's happening?' I asked.

Saul put both hands on his hips. He looked for a moment like a red-faced superhero. 'Getting out. Dis-charge. See you suckers later.' His chipped-front-tooth smile was wider than I'd ever seen it. 'Back to my life and my girl.'

'Saul,' I said. 'That's great.'

Alex dug his hands into his hoodie pocket. 'They're considering reducing his olanzapine because of the sedative effects.'

Saul kissed his teeth. 'About fuckin' time too.'

Behind them, a man in a Slipknot T-shirt was walking at pace towards us. Every muscle in his body looked gripped with fury. I watched, my chest constricting, as he swerved into his bedroom and slammed the door so hard it bounced back open off the frame. We watched him stumble over to a heavy chair, raise it in the air and smash it into the wall with a splintering howl.

'Shit!' Alex said.

We grabbed at the alarms around our necks as the man smashed again and again.

Beside us, Saul was laughing. 'Do it!' he yelled. 'Do it!' His body rocking in mirth as two nurses rushed past us and into the room, wrestling the man to the floor, his limbs thrashing.

Other patients had appeared, crowding the door and pushing into us. As we tried to drive them back, Ray emerged from the sea of faces, her arms in the air like a high diver. 'Out!

Out!' she said, sliding past us into the room and shutting the bedroom door forcefully. The sound of metal in the lock.

I looked at Alex, my heart thumping, and felt an empty, dreamlike suspension. 'Shit,' I said.

He looked redder than before, but calmer than I felt. He nodded. 'Shiiit.'

Beside us, Saul was still laughing. His reaction seemed abrasive now, unkind.

'Saul,' I pleaded. 'Don't.'

Saul stopped cold, looking at me with an unbroken, mute stare. He turned and walked away from us, his broad back disappearing into another room. A muddy guilt washed through me, twisting into my stomach. In that moment we were reminded of the rift between us, our impulsive actions enshrining our allegiance.

Fuad hadn't been sleeping well; there were dots of yellow at the corners of his eyes and his shirt had a stain on the breast. He smiled at me weakly, raising a hand as I walked into the beehive where he was sat eating a Pot Noodle. The ward seemed hotter and closer than it had moments before, and I wiped at my face with my sleeve.

'I know,' he offered. 'This isn't the staff room.'

I shrugged.

'So,' he began, his voice weary, 'a young woman called Dionne is here again.' He brought the plastic pot to his mouth and drained the liquid, before throwing the container into the bin. 'Twenty-four years old,' he continued, looking at the floor.

He paused and was silent for a moment.

'She's been admitted for swallowing razors,' he said. 'She was in for something similar before when one of her sisters died from a drug overdose. Then her brother tried to hang himself, I think.'

'Jesus,' I said, unthinkingly.

'Oh, it gets worse,' he said, rubbing at the hollow of his cheek. 'Her father's described as violent, very abusive. She's got a fresh bruise on her forehead from him throwing a bottle at her. She said she was concussed. There's also a history of rape documented in her notes.'

Gabe, the nurse from the ECT suite, walked into the beehive. His greased hair shining. He looked past me, to Fuad. 'Oof,' he said, sitting down. 'Another returner.'

Fuad's face remained static. I watched, trying to read his reaction to this man, while Gabe rearranged his feet on a table.

'I just tried to assess her,' he continued, doodling on a notepad. 'But she didn't want to talk to me – said she didn't want to talk to a *man*.'

I nodded. This made sense after hearing about her past.

'Yeah,' Fuad replied. 'She has a history of abuse by men.'

'Yeah, well.' Gabe shrugged. '*I'm* not going to abuse her though, am I? She's picking and choosing – it will be an ongoing issue in her life. *Very PD.*'

Again. *Personality disorder.* A diagnosis which seemed to be used as an insult. I looked out through the glass front and into the hallway, trying to control myself.

Gabe stood up and walked past me towards the door. He opened it and poked his head out. 'Why's she in the bathroom so long?' he said, laughing to himself. 'PD! They love themselves.'

THE BEDROOM

Another nurse appeared outside the door. 'Oh, Gabe,' she chuckled. 'Got yourself another case of *attention-attention-look-at-me*, have you?'

I left Fuad in the room and went to look for the consultant-in-charge. To my disappointment, I found Dr Oxley in the office.

'The new admission, Dionne, has asked not to speak to Gabe,' I said. 'She doesn't feel comfortable speaking to a man.'

The doctor's face remained characteristically blank. 'Probably because Gabe is putting in boundaries with her and she wants things how she wants them,' he said, knocking a pile of paper into shape on the table. 'Wants it *her way*.' He looked up. 'Just tell him to go back anyway and assess her. You can go with him if you like.'

I left the room, feeling like I wanted to punch something.

Back in the beehive, I told Gabe that we'd been told to go together. He looked peeved.

'Stay behind me, though,' he grunted. 'Don't get too involved. I'm not having her manipulating me.'

We walked together to Dionne's bedroom. Behind a propped-open door, a slight girl sat up in bed under the starched blanket, her hair bunched messily into two balls on top of her head. There was a raggedy teddy bear beside her, its face squashed and sad.

Gabe sat down on the chair near her bed. She looked at him before starting to sob, curling over to hide her face in her pillow.

'Stop crying,' Gabe said. 'It's *not good* to cry.'

Dionne looked up. 'You're rude,' she said, 'and you're stupid.'

*

I followed Gabe back into the office as he looked for the doctor. We found him chewing on the end of a pencil. Gabe explained what had happened.

'She sounds manipulative to me,' Dr Oxley replied, taking the pencil out of his mouth. 'Constant splitting; deciding if staff are worthy of her attention or not.'

Gabe was nodding.

'Lots of tattoos too, did you see them?' he said to me, gesturing to his arm. 'That's often a sign of PD.'

I glared at him.

Dr Oxley scribbled something in a leather notebook. 'Hmm.' He flicked the pencil against the pad. 'Anything from the notes last time?'

Gabe was silent.

'Her father's very abusive,' I offered. 'And she lost her sister recently.'

Gabe pinched his lips, his memory jolted. 'Oh yeah, a good relationship with her mum and a bad one with her dad, I remember. *So PD.*'

The doctor looked up. 'When was the death of her sister?'

'Over two years ago, I think,' Gabe replied. 'A *long time.* Too long for all this. Definite PD traits.' He laughed in my direction. 'Honestly.' He shook his head knowingly. 'You should join one of the group therapy sessions – *everyone* in there is PD. You'll get a crash course in whining.'

Dr Oxley was scribbling again. 'A short-term admission here will provide some respite from the home environment,' he said. 'Which seems to be exacerbating her problem.'

Exacerbating? I swallowed hard.

'But,' he continued, 'as you said, it sounds like textbook PD to me.'

As Gabe and I left the office, I asked how he could tell she wasn't suffering from complex PTSD considering the extent of her trauma. It was a diagnosis I'd only recently encountered, and was subsequently amazed at how infrequently it was spoken about. I thought back to Uma, of how close we came to missing her abuse and diagnosing her as psychotic. A diagnosis which would instantly bring into question her ability to narrate her experiences reliably.

'Oh,' he said, 'you can *fake* having PTSD. You can often just tell by looking – wait.' We stopped outside Dionne's bedroom and peered in. She was sitting in a chair with a book. 'See her posture? She doesn't have PTSD. You're always sitting up and alert with PTSD, not hunched back and chill.'

*

Complex post-traumatic stress disorder is more recently delineated and lesser known than PTSD. Both are said to be emotional responses to traumatic events, though PTSD usually results from a single-incident trauma, whereas C-PTSD arises as a response to continued, repeated or multiple forms of trauma, such as chronic sexual, emotional and/or physical abuse or neglect. It is also more commonly seen in people who experience trauma during earlier stages of development, or whose trauma relates to a care giver or guardian.

Trauma as the origin of mental and emotional distress was unacknowledged until the study of 'shell shock' in Vietnam

War veterans, and following this, PTSD was first outlined in the 1980 edition of the so-called psychiatric bible *The Diagnostic and Statistical Manual of Mental Disorders* (the 'DSM').

Both diagnoses are arguably still anomalies within psychiatry. They go some way to acknowledging traumatic and distressing life experiences as the reason for a profound psychological reaction. *It's not you or your body's fault*, these diagnoses seem to say, *it's what's happened to you*. Interestingly, such diagnoses seem to cultivate more compassion within staff, which impacts the quality of care given and type of treatments offered, diversifying more readily towards psychological and social support.

However, getting a diagnosis of C-PTSD will depend on a clinician's acknowledgement of what 'counts' as trauma, and their ability to assess a person who will likely not yet have words to recognize their suffering. As a result, extensive relational trauma is frequently missed, with distressed people instead given a label of personality disorder. This controversial diagnosis, despite many attempts to rebrand it, still carries a heavy stigma, even within the services which are meant to be caring for you. It can be weaponized against your pain and distress, your wants and needs. Your personality is *disordered*: what's wrong is *you*.

*

I searched the ward for Fuad and found him in the kitchen counting out stock.

'I know, *I know*,' he said, his face dejected. 'I just need some quiet time away from everyone...'

I sat next to him, a stack of sliced white bread in front of me on the counter, and told him about Gabe's assessment of Dionne. He made an exasperated noise.

'That guy,' he said. 'Makes me want to throw something at him.' He squatted and began piling loaves into the cupboard. 'I think a diagnosis of PTSD – especially C-PTSD – is often avoided. Or any kind of acknowledgement that they've been through something traumatic, really. Because then they have to be referred for psychotherapy, and the waiting lists are ridiculous. I mean months, years. And a lot of patients are told they're *too complex for therapy*, which feels like a bull excuse to make the waiting lists shorter.'

Fuad shut the cupboard but stayed squatting, staring vacantly into the shiny metal.

'Too complex?' he replied to himself, his voice noticeably brittle. 'Last week, a patient got rejected by the psychology team. So – she's been raped, there's incest in her childhood, domestic violence in her adulthood . . . What do I turn round and say to her? "Sorry, you're too messed up for therapy"?' He covered his eyes with his hand. 'No, I'm sorry, but psychology in most hospitals is bad, to be honest. Even when they get to the end of the list they only get sixteen sessions or something.'

He stood up and started mumbling. 'I gotta get out of here . . . gotta leave . . .' I watched Fuad bustle around the kitchen, opening doors at random, wiping his hands on his trousers repetitively. *Will this be me in a few years?* I wondered. *Trapped by my own sense of hopelessness?*

Later, I found him tapping furiously at a computer. He ushered me over.

'Have a look here,' he said, pointing at the screen. 'When Dionne came in she was on aripiprazole, an antidepressant . . . it's not written which one . . . oh yeah, sertraline, and procyclidine. When the consultant saw her, he started her on another antipsychotic called quetiapine.' He jabbed at the word on the screen. 'Why have they put this girl on two antipsychotics? She's already having to take procyclidine because of the side effects. There *must* be something else we can do.'

I watched him finish writing a note detailing her side effects, a nerve twitching in the curve of his temple. I thought of Dionne. So young, so desperate to escape her life. A life we were sending her right back into. Treating *her* as the problem, as the one who needed fixing.

I slipped out of the office and found Alex on fifteen-minute check duty. He was using Fuad's clipboard.

'All right?' he said, scratching his beard.

I walked with him.

'Not very all right,' I said.

He looked at me knowingly.

'One sec.' Alex paused and peered through the small, square glass panel in a bedroom door. 'Just need to . . .'

The patient from the earlier chair incident had his back to us in the room, bassy music pounding out from a tiny speaker. His trousers were pulled to his knees and his pallid bottom mooned out below his black T-shirt. His right arm pumped back and forth furiously. He was yelling as he pumped: 'CAN'T . . . FUCKIN' . . . CAN'T . . . FUCK . . .'

'Oh . . .' Alex flushed slightly, then grinned.

'Ah,' I heard myself say.

'Shall we . . . come back later?'

THE BEDROOM

Fuad was walking towards us. 'Hey,' he said to me, 'have you got a moment?'

'Sure,' I said, moving away from Alex, who tipped his head in acknowledgement.

'So, this is what I'm going to do.' Fuad was walking faster than usual, his face animated. 'I'm finding Dr McCulloch *now*, and I'm demanding, *demanding* that she reassesses Dionne and overrules Dr Oxley. She won't like it, but damn it, I think we're screwing up that girl's life even more than it already is, and I won't – *won't* – be a part of it.'

I resisted the urge to hug him, my heart aching with appreciation.

Later that evening, Fuad was in the beehive. I joined him at the computer. He looked drained. Outside, a young man wearing a beanie over his long hair gesticulated at us through the glass. I got up to open the door.

'Howzit, boss,' he said in a South African accent. 'Can I tell you something?' He peered around before pointing indiscreetly at a health care assistant further down the hall. 'That man,' he said, still pointing, 'pushed me into my bedroom door last night and told me to *shut up*. I was telling him I was suicidal and needed to talk to someone, and he just kept sitting there playing a game on his phone.' He put his arm down and shrugged. 'So, I put my T-shirt round my neck. *That* got his attention.'

Fuad scooted his chair across the floor so the man could see him. 'Sorry, Scott,' he said softly.

Scott nodded at him.

'We'll tell the manager.'

'Thanks, boss.' Scott saluted and walked away.

I shut the door and sat down next to Fuad.

'Who are we going to tell?' I asked.

Fuad looked at me, his eyebrows arching. 'Well,' he said, 'that kid has a diagnosis of PD, among other things. No one's going to listen. They'll say he invents things, that he's attention-seeking. And I think I've used up all my protest cards for the week now without getting myself into trouble.'

Fuad put a finger in his mouth and pulled at a nail. I had thought that the pressure to remain in staff's favour was only mine as a student, but perhaps qualified staff had to walk this uncomfortable line too.

'But, *does* he invent things?' I asked.

Fuad tilted his head thoughtfully. 'Well, I mean, yesterday he told me he's working undercover for the police.'

'Oh,' I said. 'But, does he believe that, or . . .'

'Good question.' Fuad crossed and uncrossed his legs. His body seemed jumpy suddenly, in a way I'd not seen before. He pushed his sleeve up his arm. 'The consultant has decided that *no*, he doesn't fully believe it. Otherwise he'd probably have a diagnosis of schizophrenia. I couldn't tell you exactly why he came to that decision. I'm pretty sure the consultant hates the kid, which – I'm sorry to admit – often plays a part in a PD diagnosis. Scott's also got a really bad benzo addiction, which gets staff's backs up.'

I'd noticed this peculiar contradiction; if patients *requested* benzodiazepines, staff seemed irritated and would often withhold the drug, scolding their 'drug-seeking behaviour' or 'addiction'. It made no sense to me on a ward where 90 per cent of the patients were prescribed long-term benzodiazepines.

THE BEDROOM

'Isn't he prescribed them?' I asked.

Fuad grimaced. 'Oh yeah,' he said. 'I don't really know what they expect to happen if you put people on the drug in the first place. A nurse friend of mine raised a concern about Scott's medication the last time he was here, and someone put in a complaint about her. I'm pretty sure it was Dr Oxley.'

I shook my head, dumbfounded.

'Scott was one of the people I put forward for psychotherapy, actually. He was inducted into a gang as a child in South Africa, his level of trauma is immense. Even then the referral didn't get anywhere. I think it's because people assume he's lying.'

Gabe walked into the room, tucking his shirt roughly into his jeans. 'Who?' he asked, turning to Fuad with a pinched expression.

'The South African kid,' he answered. 'One of yours?'

I spun round to the computer and key-searched 'Childhood' in Scott's file.

Gabe scanned the whiteboard where patient names and details were scribbled into columns in red. 'Oh, yeah,' he said, as if he'd forgotten. '*That* guy. He's mine.'

'There are some notes about his dad here,' I said, indicating the screen. 'He said something happened to him when he was seven. He calls his dad a *very bad man*. Ran away to live with his grandma at one point, before being in a gang. It says here that he refuses to see his dad when he comes to visit.'

Gabe looked at me impassively. 'I've met his dad, he's a very caring man – his son's mentally ill, early onset eight or nine years old.'

I looked back, feeling emboldened by having Fuad beside

me. 'But this psychology entry says something happened to him in the family home when he was seven,' I said. 'Something to do with his dad. That he can't talk about it. That he lived with his grandma and wouldn't go back home.'

'Yes.' Gabe yawned. 'He's *mentally ill.*'

Fuad looked at me, and I felt my face darkening.

'Shouldn't we try to find out if something happened?' I said. 'Maybe it would . . . help if he had counselling? Or some kind of support to—'

Gabe snorted. 'Living with other family is normal in *those* countries.' His voice was sharper now. 'Things are more family-oriented and all that.'

'Ah, of course!' Fuad said, leaning forward, his voice sour with sarcasm. He turned to me. '*See what I mean?*'

Gabe, oblivious, had opened a bag of crisps and was inspecting a particularly big one. 'Anyway,' he said to the crisp, 'we're all counsellors. Counselling is just *talking.*' He put the crisp in his mouth and it crunched into the silence. 'That Dionne girl is one of mine now,' he added. 'Might do a bit of counselling on her later.'

Ray appeared at the door. She smiled at me but her body looked stiff. 'Can we have a quick chat?'

'Sure,' I said. Something about her manner made me worry.

'Ooh,' Gabe said after she left. 'You're in trouble.'

I nodded to Fuad, who wore a puzzled expression, and followed Ray to the office.

She sat down and smiled again, clasping her hands together. The office chair rotated slowly.

'So,' she began, 'nothing to worry about at all. I just wanted

THE BEDROOM

to chat as . . . some people have told me that our student asks a lot of questions.' Her mouth sounded dry.

'Oh,' I replied, tucking my hands into my lap. 'As in *too many* questions?'

She nodded. 'I told them some people learn that way.' She paused. 'But yes, best to look things up yourself, and ask *some* questions.' She pushed her glasses up the bridge of her nose.

'So,' I summarized carefully, 'only ask *some* questions, but not others.'

Ray tilted her head. 'Yes. Better to learn by watching what others do, imitate what you see.'

I could feel confusion and anger building in me. I bit the side of my cheek. 'OK.'

Ray clasped her hands together. 'Lovely,' she said, smiling again. 'That's all good then.'

I wanted to yell at her, and dug my fingernails into my hand to stop myself.

'I was going to ask,' I said, slowly, 'who do I pass a patient complaint on to?'

Ray narrowed her eyes.

Was I retaliating? Was I trying to hurt her with this question?

'Oh?' she said.

'A patient told me and Fuad that an HCA pushed him into a door and told him to shut up.'

I watched Ray swallowing. She threaded and unthreaded her fingers.

'The thing is,' she began, 'you're a good nurse - I can tell that already. You care a lot, you spoil the patients even. But with certain situations, you have to be careful what you say and ... always assume the best of the staff, otherwise people won't want to work with you.'

I felt the air knocked out of me. I was dreaming. This wasn't really happening. I looked at her, unable to answer.

'Trust me,' Ray continued. 'We need nurses like you, and we want you sticking around. But there are patients who, well, there are a lot of unwell people whose testimonies are very unreliable, let's say.' She paused, peering at me.

I dug my nails in harder.

'Oh,' she continued, 'I know that some of our staff are less ... *charitable* than they should be. But there are some patients who are very difficult to work with, and people work very hard here.'

I must have been doing something noticeable with my face, because she leant towards me.

'Trust me,' she said, again. 'Give it time. You'll find there are some patients you won't like working with either, for whatever reason. Some who will make it challenging for you to remain so generous.'

I thought about the patients on the ward, shuffling through their faces like a deck of cards. Towards the end of the pack, a face blurred. Jack.

'He's done it again ...'

A health care assistant was dragging a large plastic bag of soiled laundry out of a bedroom, his face puckered and colourless.

'That's the last time I'm cleaning it up, I'm telling you,' he said. 'It's someone else's turn.'

I was standing in the day area, helping with the breakfast

queue. A few patients were already sitting in silence, bleary-eyed, spooning sugar-laced cereal into their mouths. Several others were standing waiting to be served. Suddenly, the thick smell of faeces filled my nostrils.

I turned round. Jack was standing behind me, his eyes dull, his mouth grinning in my direction. Ray appeared in the doorframe, waving her arms.

'Jack! Jack! Can you go and change straight away, please? Now.'

Jack gurgled and rocked on to one leg haphazardly. With his back to me, I heard him speak for the first time.

'Yeaah, yeaah, ma'am, OK, ma'am,' he drawled in a thick Scottish accent.

A brown smear climbed up the back of his hospital pyjamas. Two men in the queue noticed it and started yelling.

'Nasty!'

'You dirty fucker!'

'Aaaaahhh,' retorted Jack, dragging himself towards the hallway, dispersing the small puddle of urine that had collected around his bare feet.

I asked around the ward about Jack. Did this happen often? When did it start? Why would he do that? Nurses shrugged. He'd been night-soiling for the entire time he'd been on the ward, they said, who knows why? He used to be a heroin and crack addict. Or, maybe it was a dirty protest?

There was something about Jack that made me avoid him as much as possible. He seemed to sense my disquiet and would lean towards me, so close I could feel his breath on my cheek. I would back away, saying something about *personal space*, attempting to remain polite, to reassure him that

I could continue talking, while inside I was running off down the hall and showering vigorously, as if his proximity soiled my skin.

Jack talked in whispers. Elongated, breathy whispers that were difficult to follow. His abstruse incoherence somehow drew me in. After a few false starts in conversation across the week, I found him in his bedroom. He was sat on the end of his bed, his upper body curling forward, his hands, like something detached from him, rhythmically, mechanically rubbing circles around his knees. He looked up as I moved into the doorframe and watched me silently.

'Hi, Jack,' I said, smiling. Trying to look relaxed, feeling anything but relaxed.

Despite his bedroom door being wide open, it was as if the space was hermetically sealed from the rest of the ward; the air felt thicker, staler, the stench of ammonia mixed with a synthetic cleaning perfume. I stepped backwards, my breath shallowing.

'Jack,' I said, 'I wondered if we could talk . . .'

Sat in his bedroom, something about him was different. He seemed slighter, younger. He nodded rapidly, keenly. A movement I'd never seen him make before.

I took a small step forward, knowing I shouldn't go further but wanting to give us some sense of privacy. The ammonia knocked into me again.

'Jack,' I began, 'can you tell me what—'

'Jack!' He turned sharply to his left, his voice raised wildly as he shouted into the air. 'Stop!' I watched his head rotate back to me, his eyes sunk deep into their hollows. 'Jack says I'm a *naughty boy*.'

I felt gripped by a kind of horror, as Jack's face contorted into an unreadable mess. His body collapsed inwards, as if trying to disappear.

'You are my *best naughty friend*, Jack,' he said, turning to his spectre again, his voice low. 'You are a *good man*.'

'Jack,' I said. I could hear my voice shaking. 'Are you . . .'

I watched as Jack's curled back reared like a snake, his face red with blood. 'I'm no one!' he yelled, spittle spraying, his voice distorted into a wrathful weapon. 'I am Jack!'

And then he was laughing, laughing into the misery of that bedroom, as I backed out slowly, my head pounding, my legs unsteady. Jack's eyes followed me, his neck locked to one side.

Jack's name was not really Jack. Jack's name was Thomas. On the whiteboard in the beehive, I found Jack's name written as 'Thomas Stevenson (Jack)'. I spent my lunch break after his outburst thinking about how best to ask Jack about Jack. I couldn't shake the feeling that we were missing something deeply important. I knew Jack had been homeless most of his life, I knew that he had been a crack-cocaine addict. I knew that he was diagnosed as schizophrenic, that his behaviour and demeanour were understood by staff to be hallucinations and nothing more, and that he was prescribed a heavy, sedating dose of antipsychotic medication, as well as a benzodiazepine and a mood stabilizer. Yet there was something about Jack – the absence behind his eyes, the disquiet he instilled.

After finishing my allocated tasks, I asked a flustered, pencil-thin nurse why Jack was so adamant to be called by that name rather than his own, and if we knew anything further. The nurse was busy checking the dates on boxes of medication, meticulously recording her findings in a tiny, barely legible script.

'Oh, I'm not exactly sure,' she said, turning over a slender white box. 'It's quite common for psychotic patients to change their name or want to be called something else – especially when they're unwell.'

'Oh, right.' I couldn't leave it there. 'Strange that he talks to someone he calls "Jack" too.'

She looked at me. 'Does he? I hadn't noticed he was calling his hallucination Jack.' Her face was momentarily bemused, then she continued with her task. 'He's probably just confused. He's taken a *lot* of drugs in his time.'

'Yeah,' I replied. 'I guess.'

The next morning, I was standing behind the front desk, signing a patient and his visiting mother out of the building, when I noticed Jack leering at us, his eyes unblinking. I saw him through the visitor's eyes: this zombie, this yellow-skinned, unwashed, salivating wreck of a man in hospital pyjamas, on the same ward as my son. *What is it we are doing with this man? What is it we are doing here at all?*

I shuddered.

'Hi Jack, how are you this morning?' I asked, sounding like a counterfeit receptionist.

Jack smiled crookedly and began hobbling towards me. The man and his mother pushed through The Door into the outside world, as Jack stopped at the desk and folded sluggishly over it. I could feel myself recoiling.

'Can I go out *too*?' he asked, holding my gaze.

Something heavy settled in my stomach. 'I . . . you know that you haven't got any leave yet, you'll have to ask the doctor for some during ward round.'

Jack's mouth was still pulled into a grin, though for a moment I thought I saw a flicker of dejection. 'Yeah,' he said, looking down at the surface of the desk.

'I'm sorry,' I offered. 'I'm sure it won't be long now.'

There was a pause.

'No one comes to visit Jack . . .' He leant further towards me, and I wiped a fleck of his spit off my cheek, my hand shaking.

Jack watched me, rocking from side to side as if blown by a breeze. I stumbled through various ideas of what to say. He looked more fragile, I thought, than he had ever done.

His mouth moved, but nothing came out. The same blank eyes were looking through me, past me.

'Sorry?' I said, leaning towards him.

His mouth moved again, and this time a tiny sound was expelled.

'Sorry, you're going to have to speak up,' I said, trying to sound as patient as I could.

He smiled, and this time the words were sharp and distinct, their viscosity coating me: 'Will. You. Suck. My. Cock?'

It was as though I could feel the neuronal pathways carrying the information around my brain, travelling from one section to the next, lighting up warning signals as it went. I could hear Dr Oxley's cautions in my head. It took several seconds before any words reached my mouth. Somehow, I managed a firm rebuke. My stomach clenched, a sour taste clinging to the back of my throat.

And then Jack was apologizing, his head low, shuffling away. With his back to me, he stopped.

'Jack, I . . .'

Jack turned, then, to look at me. His battered, sunken face suddenly frightened. Something stirred in me.

'It's OK, Jack,' I said. 'Just – don't talk to me that way. We can talk about other things.'

'No one cares about me,' he said, his eyes murky with tears. 'No one came . . .'

I felt myself nodding, willing him on, but unsure if I wanted him to continue. My hands, gripping the desk, looked ashen. He was moving towards me again, his head down.

'But Jack was a *good man*,' he murmured. 'Jack was the *best man*. Jack *helped* me. He *loved me* the most.'

'Who . . . who is Jack?' My voice came out breathy, tentative, mirroring his own.

'I am *no one*,' he said. 'Jack is a *good man*. Jack *cared for me*.'

'When did you meet Jack?'

'Hah!' He rocked backwards, his mouth open.

'Who is Jack?' I tried again.

'Jack!' he yelled. Then froze. His eyes flicked to mine. 'Jack has a shop, he said to Pa – let him come! *I'll look after him*.'

'He . . . he knew your dad? Jack was a friend of your dad's?'

'I was only small . . .'

'Yes.' I nodded, my mind churning.

He stepped forward, unsteady. 'Pa *knew* him. He *knew* what he did . . . he *didn't care*. He said Jack was a *good man* . . . the *best man*. No one came . . .'

I swallowed, my thoughts tearing through my skull. 'What did Jack do?'

THE BEDROOM

He snorted, the phlegm rattling deep down inside him. His face waxy and sheened with sweat. 'Ha! Jack looked after me . . . Jack *loved* me . . . *No one loved me* – only Jack. Jack would take me home, *only me* . . . Jack . . . he'd do things . . . *only me*.' He smiled again, his eyes like empty wells. 'Jack said he was a *good man*.' He was whispering again now, and I had to lean in closer to hear him. 'He told me he was teaching me. That he was loving me.'

A door slammed shut, someone was shouting down the hall. Two nurses bolted out of the beehive. The alarm pulsed above our heads.

Jack was laughing now, a muffled, slurred laughter that sounded like it had been through a blender. 'Jack was a good man!' he bellowed. 'I am nobody! I don't exist!' He was backing away from me, his legs stumbling over each other as he headed towards the commotion, as I tried to close the conversation safely somehow, telling him he was brave to speak about it, that we would talk again soon, that it was important to keep talking.

I see a frightened little boy, his back to me, moving away down the hall. I see a little boy, lying alone on a hard floor, sobbing, naked. Telling himself that Jack loves him, that someone loves him. I see him on the streets, his body flooded with toxins, trying to obliterate his night-terrors. I see him as he is now, an empty shell still penetrated by Jack's memory. The abuser having taken up permanent residence inside the broken body, consuming him, his domination complete. Thomas obliterated, unheard. Lost.

I spent an hour looking back through all his notes using keywords: Abuse, Childhood, Trauma. Eventually I found a report from almost nine years earlier by a trainee psychologist. A report that seemed to have been long buried and forgotten. A report that led to nowhere, to no treatment or therapy or care plan.

It began: 'Thomas explained that when he was a child, there was a powerful man called Jack whom he claims knew his family. He describes Jack as a much older man, and that he was forced to give him sexual favours in return for being helped.

'Is Jack a delusion arising from Thomas's schizophrenia?' the psychologist speculated, the investigation left there and forgotten.

My whole body was aching with tension, my head dull and muted by a throb that refused to shift. I re-read the last line again and again.

I needed air. I needed to be away.

I stood up and made my way into the hallway. From the corner of my eye I could see Alex waving, trying to get my attention. I pretended I hadn't seen him. *He's stopping me being invisible*, I thought. *I want to be invisible*.

I pushed my way through The Door, past the empty reception area and buzzed out of the main entrance. The expanse of dark sky above me felt womb-like, calming. I breathed in, savouring the sharp chill of air stinging my nostrils, and hugged my arms around my chest.

'Freezing, right?' a woman's voice rose behind me.

I turned into a cloud of cigarette smoke. 'Yeah,' I said. Disappointed at the intrusion.

'I love winter though,' she continued, her shoes clacking on the concrete as she walked towards me.

The woman was two heads taller than me, in heels, a leather skirt and a yellow shoulderless top. The cigarette in her hand was coated in red lipstick. She smiled and waved like a young girl.

'Forgot to bring any other clothes with me, didn't I?' she said, tugging at the hem of her top. 'The shits pulled me out too quick, didn't let me pack a proper bag.'

I smiled, unable to muster the energy to say anything.

'At least they're letting me out for cigs now, though,' she added, taking a final drag before stubbing it out on the wall beside us.

I nodded. Wishing I was alone, but grateful, too, for her persevering friendliness.

'It's a fuckin' inferno on my ward.' She smiled and flicked the butt into the flower bed behind her. 'Why do you people always put the heating on so high?'

I shook my head and laughed. It was true – why was it always a fucking inferno on the ward?

The woman laughed loudly. '*Idiots*,' she said, incredulous. 'The lot of them.'

As she said this, I noticed she had begun feeling around under her skirt. Now she dropped to a casual squat, her knees jutting out on either side of her like a crab. Her hand between her legs, she acknowledged my confused expression.

'One moment,' she said.

Her hand now appeared to be up and inside her. She pouted her lips momentarily, her shoulders rising. There was a pause, then her hand reappeared holding a crumpled, glistening box of Marlboro Reds.

'There!' she said, standing up triumphantly.

I watched her open the box and take out a pristine cigarette. She placed it between her red lips.

'I have to hide them up there otherwise it's always *GILL! YOU GOT A FAAAG?* All the fuckin' time. Now everyone leaves my fags alone because I tell them they're up my pussy.'

Later, I found Davina, the psychologist from my first day on the ward, hunched up in front of a computer. I explained everything Jack had told me. As she listened, her body seemed to wilt, though her face remained taut and disfigured in something like revulsion.

'OK, *OK*,' she said, looking away. 'I'll talk to him and see what he says.'

I was helping in the day area, cleaning up plates, when Davina appeared, her normally pristine hair ruffled, her jumper pulled out of shape. She stopped in front of me. 'Just to let you know,' she said, fidgeting with a lock of hair, 'I'm going to try and talk with him now.' She pulled at her sleeve. The skin around her fingernails looked raw.

I watched her gesture to Jack to sit on one of the chairs before positioning herself opposite him on a sofa. She leant forward on her elbows and adjusted her body numerous times before settling on a humped posture. He looked at her vacantly, wiping his mouth on his pyjama top. There were several other patients in the room, each oblivious to one another, nursing their own wounds.

I busied myself at the coffee station, moving plastic cups and torn sugar sachets into the bin. Behind me, I could hear Davina's voice but couldn't make out what she was saying. I imagined that the pauses were filled with his breathy words, though with my back to them I couldn't be sure. Davina's voice again, and then an unusually long pause. I stopped moving, straining to hear.

Then her voice rang out, louder this time: 'Can you . . . just say that again, Jack?' It sounded thin, as though she hadn't taken enough air.

I turned round. There, sitting in that chair, I saw Thomas, not Jack. Poker-straight, his face pink and resolute, altered, new. Thomas, filling that bleak room. Calling out, his body demanding to be seen, to be heard. Refusing to be silent any more. He was Thomas, and this was his story.

'Hey, Madam Jailer.' Saul was beside me by The Door, a tatty backpack slung over one shoulder.

'Saul!' Relief washed over me. He was grinning again, and there was a small gold hoop in his ear.

He noticed me looking at it. 'Got all my shit back too,' he said, rubbing the ring between his large fingers. 'Didn't realize how much I missed my fuckin' shoelaces.'

I had a sudden flash of our first meeting, by this same door several months earlier. I had been frightened then, of his otherness. Consumed by fictions of who he and I and all of us were.

'Take care out there,' I said, feeling a heaviness rising in me. It caught me off guard, and I swallowed, silencing myself. *I can't cry*, I thought. *What would it mean to cry right now?* I was afraid that if I started, everything would rush at me, an obliterating avalanche. And Saul was getting out – that was good, wasn't it? He would be somewhere better than here. I wanted to believe that for Saul and for all the patients, this place was merely a glitch before things brightened exponentially ahead; like an explosive dawn, blasting away the nightmares of the evening before.

'High-five?' he said, his hand hovering in the air.

5

The Day Area

ALEX'S SPORADIC DAYS ON THE ward had come to an end, and without the interruption of his familiar face my submersion in the ward deepened. It felt both lonely and freeing – released from the precariousness of our camaraderie, but waking from the lull of that semblance of safety was harsh. Alone, I felt the driving impetus towards uniformity more acutely, the exhaustion of constant obstructed enquiry.

The day area was the biggest open space on the ward, sandwiched between the two locked rooms labelled 'The Chill-Out' and 'The Get-Together'. One corner of the area backed on to the shuttered kitchen, the adjacent space swallowed by four synthetic dining tables (too heavy to pick up) and chairs (still throwable). The other half resembled a soft play centre, with heavy, primary-coloured plastic sofas made to be unbreakable and unself-harmable. Opposite the sofas, a large TV entombed in a smash-proof box was bolted to the floor. It was a space used for queueing and eating in silence, for staring blankly at the TV. A place where each patient's isolation was sharply delineated. The walls were bare, with one reinforced window. A pool table without any balls or cues had been pushed into a corner, retired more than six months previously after a man had used a cue to try and break the window. The green felt was now a canvas for nail-scratched protests: FUCK YOU and GIVE IT BACK. Occasionally the area would hold a psychology group or host a visiting therapist conducting a workshop, but for the largest portion it remained an empty shell. An uncanny refraction of adult life that invited regression: to smear and fling and shriek.

Finlay stood in the day area, a battered suitcase on the floor beside him. As I walked past, he lifted his flat cap and rubbed his wiry white head of hair. At ninety, he was the ward's oldest resident and notably drew much affection from the staff. 'Lovely to see you this morning, Finlay!' nurses would exclaim as they passed him. He would look on after them, bemused, shaking his head as if they were naughty school children.

Finlay was tiny, in both height and physique. His back was bent almost double, his feet disfigured by fierce bunions. Yet he remained constantly on the move and hardy as a bull. Mostly he remembered the people around him but lost his sense of time and place, his mind creating elaborate yet mundane worlds that wholly consumed him. Often he was at a bus stop watching the hum of traffic pass. He would wave to invisible passers-by, stare at invisible screens for arrival updates, instructing himself in a lilting Barbadian accent to 'collect things' to 'pack up for home', a dog-eared timetable clenched in his fist. Other days he'd spend hours delicately taking apart an invisible object at a table, or attempting to make space for something large to pass through the day area, ordering incredulous patients to *move their legs out the way*, and pressing his slight body fervently into the side of a sofa, somehow managing to squeak it a few centimetres across the floor. His face creased in concentration, his eyes incandescent within the folds of skin.

'He's always off somewhere,' a nurse affirmed as she passed.

There were also days when Finlay was unable to escape the vacuum between these walls. He faced this bitter reality with an armour of elbows and muttering, refusing to eat anything or speak to anyone as he paced the room, wagging his finger like a prefect. Sometimes he could be roused from this demeanour with the reminder that he loved to sing.

'Finlay has a beautiful voice!' a nurse would exclaim, patting his shoulder. 'Isn't that true?'

And then Finlay would melt, his arms falling to his sides, his face rising from the floor, eyes widening as he opened his mouth and began to sing like an old maestro.

His ad-libbed lyrics were clear and complex, as he weaved in and out of the stories from his past: down by the harbour at night, meeting beautiful girls during travels through Europe, fights with friends over lovers. Then he would stop abruptly and appear irritated. His next sentence jumbled, as if singing had temporarily disconnected the cables in his brain and wired them back all wrong. 'You and you lot to do over the place!' he'd yell at someone. His body all at an angle again, as he trudged away out of sight.

The warmth Finlay inspired in staff was both entirely explicable and curious to me. Unlike the majority of the male patients, he was small and brittle, his physique inspiring guardianship rather than fear. Yet, I also wondered if his diagnosis made him more palatable. Dementia and its related neurological diseases still sit – though contested – within psychiatry. These conditions are notable for their categorical visibility within scans and tests: they are *known*. They afflict us at particular ages with regularity. Generally, they do not sneak up on us unawares, or consume our children. We feel we have some grip on dementia, some power over it, and so perhaps on the people within its clutches.

Before the gradual fragmentation of his mind, Finlay had worked with his hands, building and shaping and mending. Now he struggled to find tasks to fill the spaces in his day, his hands, unoccupied, no longer remembering what to do.

'This needs sorting,' he would say to no one in particular.

'What do you want to sort, Finlay?' someone would ask, their tone gentle and noncommittal, as if appeasing a petulant toddler.

He would pause, confused by the response.

'Home,' he would say firmly, and then look around perplexed by his own answer, trying to catch someone's eye – perhaps they could bring clarity?

Some days Finlay would stand in the day area for an hour, repeating this couplet of phrases. Until finally, disheartened, his mind would take him elsewhere.

'Lots of work,' he would say to his shoes, his speech slowing. 'Anything to . . . clean?'

Staff shuffled past, their eyes avoiding his.

After watching him for several days, I asked a nurse if I could give him some cups to wash. We can make it an activity,

THE DAY AREA

I suggested. I was told it wasn't possible due to health and safety regulations.

Instead, Finlay was prescribed the antidepressant sertraline.

As it neared the time of the drug's expected effect, to my surprise I noticed a change. An energy within him, more smiles, a swing to his walk. Staff nodded to one another knowingly, reminding Finlay frequently how *happy* he looked. They took him on the shop-run to get milk. His face burning with pride as he passed the cartons to the kitchen staff.

'You're very welcome!' he beamed.

But as the days rolled on, Finlay resumed his position at the day area bus stop. He continued to ask for tasks, his confusion worsening. Staff seemed disappointed in him. They stopped taking him on the shop-run.

One morning I found Finlay dressed entirely in black, sat in a solitary chair positioned in front of the day area window. He was motionless, staring into the falling rain. There was a tear on his cheek. A health care assistant noticed me watching and leant over, whispering in my ear, 'He thinks he's going to his daughter's funeral today.'

I watched for some minutes, unsure what to do. It seemed an awful thing to sit with, alone.

My thoughts were bouncing about, trying to find a hold. What was the best thing to do here? Indulge the delusion? Counter it? The weight of the scene seemed too bottomless to comply with, so much more distressing than his usual realities. I wanted to pull him out into the present, even if that present was here.

'Finlay,' I said, 'are you OK?' I crouched down beside his chair.

He didn't move, his face resolute with grief.

I put my hand on his arm. The touch seemed to stir something in him.

'Is the bus coming?' he said, his voice cracked with pain.

'Finlay,' I said again. 'What's happened?'

Finlay told me his youngest daughter had died. That he had to get the bus on time. 'Where's the right stop? Can you show me the way?' he asked, wiping his face with a handkerchief. 'I can't find my home.'

For hours Finlay went round in circles. He sat at the window, then looked in vain for an exit. Tears weaving through his crumpled skin. A few nurses tried to convince him that everything was OK.

'Your daughter's at work!' they said as they swept past. 'She's totally fine!'

Finlay didn't hear them.

I tried a number of times to talk with him. He told me, *thank you*, but he needed to be alone right now. So I watched from afar, like a bystander at an accident. Fascinated, disturbed, entirely impotent.

Then it came to me. Nothing miraculous. Nothing particularly clever. But, maybe, I could call his daughter.

When I finally got through to Alesha and explained, she sighed down the phone. 'Oh dear,' she breathed, sounding tired. I could hear voices and commotion in the background.

'Finlay,' I said, holding the phone out towards him.

He looked at me, perplexed, his reddened eyes squinting. He held the phone as if something might spring from it, before pressing it carefully to his ear.

'Alesha?'

Pause.

'That you, baby?'

Pause.

'What happened to you? How'd you fall down?'

Pause.

'How can you be at work? Why aren't you in a hospital?'

Pause.

'But you're OK? They say you'll be OK?'

Finlay was crying again, but the tears seemed lighter, weightless.

'Praise God!' he said, cupping the phone like a precious jewel. 'She's going to be OK! My baby is OK!'

Every bristle on his face seemed to be shining. It was the closest I've ever come to seeing joy fully comprehended, fully realized in corporeal form.

'*Thank you*,' he said, clasping my hand urgently as my breath shortened, my heart knocking hard against my ribcage. 'You will stay friendly with her, won't you? Make sure she's OK?'

And in that single moment I too was wholly consumed. As though there was nothing else in the world, nothing more real than this man, than this place.

Within the hour, Finlay was clearing space in the day area again, the look of recognition in his eyes gone.

A nurse moved over to me. 'He'll be right back where he started now,' she said. 'Hard to keep up trying with him.'

I nodded. It was true.

Though, perhaps the only way through, I mused as I watched Finlay pushing at a heavy table, was to exist from moment to moment. To relinquish the goal of progress and seek transitory release. Fleeting connection. The embrace of going nowhere. Maybe that was OK, maybe that was enough.

As I turned around, I noticed today's allocated two-to-one health care assistants leaning casually against the wall, one playing a game on his phone, the other watching a soap opera on the TV. They looked up and smiled vaguely in my direction, before their eyes drifted over to a stooped, mumbling man circling the dining table Finlay was trying to shift. Neither man acknowledged the other. I watched Kumar finish rounding it, and then do the same with each table, before heading for the open door. One of the health care assistants groaned as they both traipsed after him.

'Where are we going *now*?' one laughed.

'My feet are killing me, no joke,' said the other.

Kumar was also diagnosed with dementia. Though unlike Finlay, he was never left alone, even when sleeping. Two staff were assigned to follow him closely at all times.

'He can be really violent, right out of nowhere,' Ray had warned me. 'So, don't get in his way.'

Kumar had just turned sixty-four and had advanced, early-onset dementia. In five years he'd gone from a robust, successful businessman to a frail, incoherent man wearing an incontinence pad. He now spent his days wandering tirelessly, his unfocused eyes still warm and learned, his smooth hair framing his handsome black-and-white-movie-star face.

He would be in assisted living, I was told, if it wasn't for his violence. A violence that would burst from him whenever his incontinence pad was being changed. It had resulted in one health care assistant with a broken nose, one with a sprained finger, and another with a slapped face.

'Kumar!' One of the assistants was steering him back into the day area. 'Let's go *here*, OK?' He navigated Kumar over to a sofa and positioned him there. 'Yes, *good*.'

Kumar stood up. He was sat back down. He stood up again and was coaxed back into a seated position.

'Sit down for a little,' the HCA said. 'Let's watch this show. Yes?'

The other assistant was chuckling. 'Good luck with that.'

I watched them make several attempts to keep him there, holding his arms, telling him to *be still*, that he needed to *rest*. They managed close to five minutes before Kumar calmly overpowered them and began making his way to the door again. His eyes darting about the floor and walls, his mouth constantly working a chewing action. Both men groaned and stood up.

Just outside the doorway, I watched Kumar jolt excitedly forward, moving at pace, the men skipping after him. He stopped, bent down as if to pick up something from the floor, grasping at the air, and then stood, opening his fist to survey the emptiness quizzically.

I approached him. 'What did you see?' I asked, curious to know if he could answer me.

Kumar looked up, his eyes focused somewhere behind my left ear, humming vowels to an upbeat tune. I listened to the rise and fall of his voice. The rhythm was soothing.

'You found something there?' I tried again, wanting to make some kind of contact.

Kumar closed his eyes and smiled.

And then, suddenly, his limbs were moving towards me in a flurry.

'Kumar!' shouted one of the HCAs, lunging forward. 'Slowly! Careful!' He gripped his arm as Kumar reached my side.

The momentary tightness in my chest released. Perhaps foolishly, I realized, I wasn't afraid of this man, despite what I'd heard. My privileged naivety.

He looked straight at me now, humming his vowels, and took my hands in his. They were warm.

'Warm hands,' I said.

Kumar tilted his head, watching me. Then he brought my hands to his mouth and blew two hot breaths on them, rubbing enthusiastically. I looked at him in surprise, and he smiled, triumphant.

'Oh!' I said. 'Thank you!'

And then he was off again.

'Look!' he exclaimed in a flurry of coherence. 'Show something . . .'

I exchanged raised eyebrows with one of the assistants, who opened his mouth into an astonished O.

Kumar and I walked a few steps together back into the day area. It felt like there was real direction to his stride, real purpose. And then, he stopped. The rumbling of syllables began again.

'Kumar?' I said. 'What did you want to show me?'

He stood, motionless, his eyes roving about the room before fixing on the pool table. He pointed to it.

We moved forward together.

'This?' I asked.

Kumar reached out and smoothed the felt with his fingertips. I did the same.

'It feels nice,' I said.

Kumar smiled. It felt, somehow, like we were sharing something. Even if it was only sensation on skin.

Then he turned abruptly again, and was out of the room. Disappearing around the corner, the HCAs in his wake.

Each day, Kumar explored the ward as if for the first time. Yet, I noticed on some days he was more interactive, framing questions with a glint of recognition, of playfulness in his wandering eyes. Other days the difference was stark: he was slumped and drooling, incapable of responding to anyone. Perplexed, I read through Kumar's prescribed medication and noticed he was taking a number of sedating drugs. A medication for dementia called memantine, the antidepressant/painkiller trazodone, the antipsychotic olanzapine and two benzodiazepines: lorazepam daily, and the stronger clonazepam 'as and when required' – known as 'PRN', after the Latin pro re nata – to be given at 'the nurse's discretion'.

I found Dr McCulloch in the office. She was filling in a prescription while eating a sandwich. She gestured for me to sit down.

'Could I ask you about Kumar?' I said.

She looked up and smiled. 'Sure,' she said, frowning at what I imagined was my anxious expression. 'What's worrying you?'

I told her about his varying presentation and asked which of the medications might be causing it.

She took a bite of her sandwich and looked thoughtful. 'Well, really it could be any of them,' she said. 'I'm not fully sure how we arrived at that combination, to be completely frank, but he's a tricky one. Violence against staff is very serious, and we have to help him to be more *tranquil* somehow.'

'*Tranquil*,' I echoed, wanting her to go on.

'Well,' she said, 'if I want him to be *tranquil*, I give him a *tranquillizer*, in the form of an antipsychotic.'

Something stirred in me, surprised by her use of the word tranquillizer. 'Oh, so you're saying—'

'And,' she interrupted, 'I did add the clonazepam after that last violent incident, I'm afraid.'

'Oh.' I paused. Clonazepam was the strongest benzodiazepine and extremely sedating.

'And in combination with the tranquillizer,' she added, tapping her finger on the desk, 'that might be the culprit.'

That unexpected word again.

'I'm surprised you called the antipsychotic a tranquillizer,' I said, carefully. 'I mean, I've read about that being the original name – due to their effects. It's just not something I've heard any staff acknowledging before.'

Dr McCulloch laughed. 'Well, it's really what they are, for the most part . . . that and emotion dampeners.'

A rush of relief flooded through me. A relief at the clarity and honesty of her answers. I realized after so many months of vague responses how much I'd been hoping, longing for this.

Dr McCulloch looked away, twisting the bangle around her wrist.

'It's not an easy decision,' she continued. 'Using antipsychotics in dementia is pretty contested. It's a bit – well, more than a bit – risky. But we've got our backs against the wall with this one.'

'I had read that,' I replied. 'About it being dangerous.'

She paused.

'You know,' she said, 'it might be the clonazepam that's doing it.'

I nodded. 'OK, thanks. I'll ask the nurse on medication round if it's been given recently.'

She stood up, screwing the sandwich wrapper into a ball. 'Thanks for flagging it though.'

'Right.' I nodded. 'Thanks for your time.'

She turned again. A weak, grey light had pushed up against the window, making the room feel lifeless.

'I must say,' she began slowly. 'I had a tough time deciding whether to go into psychiatry when I was a trainee. Sometimes I'm still unsure about it.'

*

There is rigorous debate as to whether psychiatric drugs are safe or effective in managing challenging behaviours in dementia, yet they are still frequently prescribed. It's acknowledged that antipsychotic drugs may reduce aggression, but because of their severe and common side effects – excessive sedation, risk of falls, increased confusion, blood clots, stroke, even death – this is often at the expense of the person's quality of life, or of keeping them alive at all. There is an ongoing national drive by dementia charities to reduce inappropriate prescribing of antipsychotic drugs, advocating for all non-drug approaches to have been properly attempted first. However, it is thought that around two-thirds of antipsychotic prescriptions in dementia are still inappropriate, with research indicating that use of these dangerous medications could be reduced dramatically if staff were trained and supported to help individuals practically and encourage hobbies and social activities.

Despite the well-documented harms of benzodiazepines showing they are largely ineffective, not evaluated often enough to be safe, and cause fall-related injuries, pneumonia, and cognitive and coordination deterioration, these drugs are also still frequently used. As a result, care givers should always be given detailed information regarding any changes in prescription to enable the opportunity to weigh the harm/benefit ratio. Without this sharing of information, decisions belong to the staff alone.

*

The next day, an agency nurse was pushed hard against the wall as he tried to pull Kumar's trousers to his ankles to change him.

Now every day as Kumar walked, a long strand of spittle clung to his lower lip and trailed on to his T-shirt. His head folded more acutely towards his chest, his eyes staring at the floor. Some days he slept sitting up in a chair for hours.

And Kumar had been fainting. Across several days he twice fell to the ground; his eyebrow cut, his head bruised. Without warning he crumpled, his head bouncing on the linoleum.

I checked over his medication chart and saw that after the violent incident nurses had taken up their option for the discretionary (PRN) use of daily clonazepam.

I found a nurse I hadn't seen before on the medication round trolley and asked if she'd already seen Kumar.

'No,' she said, checking her list. 'But he's next.'

We walked together to the day area and found Kumar talking to himself quietly, moving up and down the room, circling tables. She opened several boxes and tipped the coloured tablets into a paper pot. She checked Kumar's drug chart, her finger hovering over the word *clonazepam*.

'Withhold if necessary,' she read aloud. 'Give if agitated.'

The nurse looked over at him, as he bent to clutch at the air near the floor, an inquisitive noise leaving his mouth.

'He doesn't seem drowsy,' she said, opening the clonazepam packet.

My stomach lurched; I could feel the heat coming from my face. *What is the meaning of agitated?* I thought. *Could the decision to sedate to a dangerous level be predicated on semantic confusion? How can a decision really be made when the staff member knows nothing of the person in front of them? Is this clonazepam preventive, punitive or merely thoughtless?*

'He's not *agitated*,' I pleaded, unable to unravel these thoughts. 'That's just how he is. He doesn't need that, he's fine – look. He's not agitated or aggressive.'

The nurse observed me expressionlessly. I was reminded, then, of my status: I was merely a student nurse, and she knew it. She continued opening the packet and retrieved a beige clonazepam tablet from the foil. She dropped it into the pot.

'Kumar?' she called out. 'Medication time.'

Later, during handover, Ray and three of the nurses discussed the impending visit of Kumar's wife.

'She'll be concerned,' one of them said. 'She'll probably get angry again. I'm not sure what to say to her.'

Ray shook her head. 'Look, she shouldn't get angry with you, that's not OK. She's only concerned about her husband being drowsy, not about staff being hit or going off sick.'

Another nurse folded her arms. 'Let *her* take him home for one day and see if she can handle it.'

Ray stood up. 'Keep the medication as it is, or up it if he hits out again. It's my responsibility to make sure you're all safe in this. Staff come first. End of story.'

Kumar's wife visited two times a week. She would sit or walk about the ward with him for hours, telling him stories, reading him books.

Today, she stood in the hallway shaking, her cheeks flushed.

'Excuse me,' she said to a nurse beside me, her voice quivering with anger. 'Has my husband been *drugged*?'

The nurse shook his head. 'No,' he said. 'He's only been given what's prescribed.'

Kumar's wife looked stricken. 'Are you sure it's . . . right?'

'Yes,' the nurse said. 'He's only getting what he needs.'

The nurse moved on.

I watched Kumar's wife, my heart racing. The word *needs* had dug into me. It was true that Kumar had hurt staff, but wasn't there something – anything – else we could do? Didn't she have the right to know that a decision to sedate him had been made, and didn't she have a right to protest this?

I asked her if she knew what medication her husband was taking and if she'd been told about the recent change. She looked at me, her eyes filled with tears, and shook her head.

'No one tells me anything here,' she said, her voice low. 'But I would like to know, *please*.'

Fuck this, I thought. I gave her a list.

The next day I searched for Dr McCulloch again, my head already throbbing. It had begun to feel almost constant, this headache. Even at home it didn't shift. I found her filling in forms in the office.

I told her about Kumar falling, the sleeping, the drooling.

'Hmm,' she said, looking at me steadily. 'I hadn't been informed. Well, I'll write off the clonazepam for a couple of days and let's see what happens.'

After two days without clonazepam, Kumar's head faced forward again. He moved, he hummed, his eyes found mine.

'Hello!' he said. 'Yes please!'

Then, something magical happened. A music therapist came to the ward. Two nurses carried in her keyboard and set it up in the middle of the day area. Patients walked past slowly, craning their necks as they tried to ascertain what was going on without conceding interest. The therapist, her head wrapped in a bright scarf, called hopefully to them to join.

Fuad entered the room with the young South African man, Scott. They both stopped beside the piano. Fuad smiled and elbowed Scott playfully.

'I think you're a bit of a musician, right?' he said.

Scott grinned. 'I'm good at karaoke,' he said, watching the therapist tinkle up and down the keys.

'Please,' she said, gesturing with her hand for him to move closer.

Scott launched into a Bon Jovi song, pretend mic in hand, the occasional leg-lunge, while staff and patients watched, clapping along. For a moment we could have been anywhere, equally trapped, equally free.

I turned round to see Kumar. Spinning to the music. His face pointed up towards the ceiling, a smile stretched clean across it.

Spotting him, Scott walked over and patted him on the shoulder. 'Boss,' he said, 'you want a go?'

Kumar shuffled around Scott's extended arm, mumbling.

'Take it to the stage,' Scott tried again.

Behind them, the therapist had started playing something familiar. 'Eleanor Rigby', I thought, recognizing the chords. Kumar lumbered towards the piano. Everyone was silent, watching him, as he stood next to the therapist, swaying, moving his arms.

'Do you remember this song?' the beaming therapist asked him as he shimmied behind her. 'Do you like the Beatles?'

'Yes!' Kumar shouted. 'Yes!'

'OK! *Wait one moment.*' She shuffled through the pages of the music book. 'I have another one here.'

The therapist began to play 'Yesterday'. The stark notes ringing out, shimmering into the gloom like jewels.

'Suddenly,' Kumar sang, his head angled towards the piano. 'Man ... used ... be.' The melody clear and unforgotten. 'Shadow ... me.' Every face in the room was mesmerized. 'I believe ... yesterday.'

I felt something in me, breaking.

*

Research outlines the many benefits of creative therapies for mental health conditions, showing decreased rates of distress and a significant impact on patients' wellbeing, self-esteem and mood. Music therapy in particular has been shown to play a substantial role in reducing the use of coerced or forced medication to control agitation and aggression. Yet, it remains notoriously difficult to quantify and prove the positive impact of these therapies in a way the medical world substantiates. So, psychiatry remains restrained in its financial investment, considering them to be peripheral rather than essential. On our ward, a creative group was offered just once or twice a week, and with granted access dependent on 'good behaviour' they were available to only a handful of patients at a time.

*

By the morning handover, I'd made my decision: I needed to see for myself. Watching Kumar grasp at the tendrils of his disappearing self and gain purchase, if only momentarily, was enough to hope that his violence could be avoided. Somewhere down the line I knew it would be too late, but now, *now* – perhaps there was another way.

I looked around the beehive. Agency staff and ward nurses were talking, their heads turning to one another. I watched them, feeling markedly alone. At some point I'd stopped looking into these faces and feeling assured.

Fuad walked in and made his way over to me. A tension released.

'Fuad!' I said. 'I'm *so glad* you're in.'

He frowned warmly, bemused by my emphatic greeting. 'Thanks,' he said.

'Can we try something together?' I asked him.

'Hah,' he laughed. 'Sure, sounds interesting.'

I turned to the day's nurse-in-charge. 'Can I help with Kumar today?' I said. 'Can I take the two-to-one duty?'

A health care assistant beamed. 'Please!' he said. 'Take my job!'

The nurse-in-charge ignored the assistant and looked at me pointedly. 'It's not safe,' she said, sitting down. 'If you, as a student, get hit then we aren't covered.'

'I can be the other two-to-one,' Fuad said, leaning forward. 'She's with me anyway this morning, and it would be a good learning opportunity. I'll make sure she stands back and watches most of the time.' He turned to me and winked comically.

'I'll stand back,' I assured the nurse-in-charge. 'I'll just watch.'

The nurse stood up again and slapped her thighs with both hands. 'Fine, fine,' she said, clearly uninterested. 'But keep at a distance.' She turned to the rest of the room. 'Will someone come and get me if anything kicks off? I'll be in the office.'

As staff filtered out, Fuad turned to me enquiringly. 'Sounds like it's you and me doing something together then.' He laughed. 'What are you planning?'

We spent the morning following behind Kumar, watching him, asking questions. Sitting with him as he gulped down water, his face screwed up as if drinking something foul. We spoke about changing his pad, what we would watch for, knowing that was the riskiest time for violence.

At around midday, Kumar started to rub at his tummy, pinch at his sides, clench his jaw. Fuad looked at me. We knew this was the moment.

'Kumar, *please*,' Fuad said gently as Kumar tried to steer away from his bedroom door. 'It will be really quick, we promise.'

I put my hand on his right arm, Fuad had his left, as we walked him in together.

Kumar was moaning now, his eyes reduced to slits within his open face.

I could feel my body shaking with adrenalin. *Was this a good idea? What was my naivety instigating now?*

As we got over to the bed, we tried to guide him into a seated position. As Kumar stepped backwards, he stumbled, gripping my wrist – hard. Fuad moved towards him rapidly, and Kumar shoved at his torso with his strong arms.

My heart leapt. My tongue sticking to the roof of my mouth. I looked at Fuad. He looked back. His eyes wide.

But something kept us talking, calmly and softly. Almost whispering as we began to unbutton his trousers and move them down his tense thighs. I watched Kumar's arm muscles flex, taut and rigid. Watched his hands ball into fists. As the trousers reached his knees, I noticed Kumar tugging at the hem of his hovering T-shirt, gripping it, stretching it towards the floor. Fuad noticed too – we looked at each other.

'I'm sorry, Kumar,' Fuad said. 'We have to take this pad off and put on another one.'

There was a groan as his hands grabbed at his T-shirt again. He stumbled backwards momentarily.

'Wait! Wait, Kumar.'

I searched the room for a towel, an item of clothing. Anything. I found a pair of shorts.

'Here,' Fuad said to Kumar as he took them from me.

As the pad slipped down, we swiftly covered his genitals with the balled-up shorts, and Kumar's tense body instantly fell limp. His arms relaxing, his breathing slowing.

He let us change him without issue.

Afterwards, the three of us sat in silence on the bed, breathing. I thought I could hear the sound of my own heartbeat. Fuad caught my eye and smiled.

'OK,' he said. 'Ready?'

We helped Kumar up, his hands still gripping the cloth shorts across his body. Carefully, we slid his trousers back to his waist, his fingers guiding ours. We left the room together.

Later that day, Fuad called Kumar's wife. He explained what had happened and told her we might have found another way. Through the receiver, I could hear her crying.

'If that's really what it is . . . *really* . . . then this could *change everything*,' she told Fuad. 'This could mean he's placed near home. That we can see him every day – he won't be miles away. That he can *leave* that dreadful place.'

Fuad sat at a computer and wrote a note for Kumar's file explaining what had happened. We talked to the health care assistants who'd previously looked after Kumar and asked what they felt had worked. Then, using this information and that day's experience, we wrote a list of 'tips' for new staff allocated to work with him.

During handover, Fuad passed the list to an agency worker

and explained to the rest of the team what we'd done. I stuck the list on the staff noticeboard.

Ray looked at us, incredulous. 'Huh,' she said, putting her hands on her hips. 'It can't really be as simple as all that, *can it?*'

Two weeks later, with no further record of violence or aggression, Kumar was relocated nearer to his family. He no longer needed to be held on a psychiatric ward.

I left that day like a firework, exploding into the darkness. *One day at a time*, I thought; perhaps that was all it took. *Just one day at a time.*

*

The next morning, by reception, I met Rashid. He was handing over a cardboard box of meticulously organized possessions. A smartphone, an expensive-looking leather wallet, a pair of earphones, two keys attached to a football pendant and a spotless baseball cap. All placed side by side, an equal width apart, as if in a display cabinet.

'Please be careful with those,' he asked the nurse. 'They're my very important things.' He smiled politely and thanked her. 'And would it be possible to have my shoes back on this ward, ma'am? I haven't been allowed to wear them upstairs. That would be very kind, thank you.'

As I watched, I became aware of something unusual about the interaction. Something unnerving. And then it hit me: he was treating this nurse as an equal; there was no frustration or animosity or despondency. He was too new to all of this.

Rashid was a nineteen-year-old Muslim man wearing a blue Adidas tracksuit, sporting a neatly shaved beard and carrying a Koran under his arm. In the wake of a surge in anti-Islamic violence around the world, Rashid had become increasingly anxious that he and his family would be attacked. Prior to being brought into the hospital he hadn't slept in days and reported feeling frightened, dazed and emotional. He had been found by police walking the streets in pyjamas, confused, reading the Koran aloud and weeping. The police had decided he needed an assessment and tried to force him into a police car. He'd refused to get in, but they insisted. Rashid tried to fight them off, and four policemen bundled him into the back and handcuffed him. As a result of this transgression he was deemed 'violent', bypassing the Acute Ward and going straight upstairs to PICU.

After four days sedated into sleep by clonazepam, Rashid was transferred down a level to our ward. That same day, Dr Oxley had assessed him and given the vague diagnosis of 'schizotypal/psychosis'. He was prescribed a continuation of twice-daily clonazepam, and the antipsychotic olanzapine.

'I feel fine now after sleeping,' he told me as we went to sit on a sofa in the day area. 'I don't have an illness, I don't need medication. I was just kinda freakin' out and stuff – the world is *crazy* at the moment. Gave me some weird insomnia and shit.'

We talked for some time about his new ward, and he watched with deep interest the other patients moving about or slumped near by. He said he felt like an anthropologist.

'I don't know,' he whispered. 'It's pretty weird here you know. What's with some of these people? They're like zombies or something!' He laughed, but his features looked strained.

Across the room, Bertie walked in. Since the reduction of his lorazepam after fainting in the sink he'd released some of the various clothing and household items from his fists, though with a jumper trailing from one hand and three different-coloured socks from the other he still looked encumbered. His dreadlocks bounced around as he moved towards one of the tables. Rashid spotted him and grinned, jumping to his feet.

'Hello, hello, brother!' he said to Bertie. 'You have awesome dreads, dude.'

Bertie stopped walking, his eyes widening in surprise. It took him several seconds to acknowledge that it was him who was being addressed so warmly. 'Heeeheee,' he responded uncertainly. 'Thanks, man.' He grinned sluggishly, but his eyes were shining.

How unusual, I thought, to see two patients conversing like friends. There was something about the ward, despite the designated communal spaces, that propelled each patient into a solitary abyss.

Rashid was now patting Bertie on the back, his face full of affection. 'Ah, mate,' he continued, pointing, 'what you got those socks for? Where you off to with those?' He laughed kindly. 'You need them all the time?'

Bertie was laughing too, his eyes moving from Rashid to his laden hands as if they were not his own.

'You gotta get some free hands going on there, man – you're dragging too much stuff for a cool guy!'

I felt myself smile; the movement of muscles like butter melting. I watched in awe as Rashid made Bertie the centre of his world, as Bertie filled with sheer glee.

From the corner of the day area, I caught sight of a nurse

striding across the room, her arms swinging beside her, her lips pulled tight.

'Hey! Hey! Rashid . . .'

The two men turned to face her. Rashid's hand froze on Bertie's back.

The nurse reached them, her chest visibly rising and falling. 'Rashid, please . . . please . . . let Bertie *be*. Give him some space.'

The two men said nothing as she removed Rashid's hand from its resting place.

I stood up. 'No, no . . . it's – they were only being friendly, just talking . . . it's all OK.' My words came out jagged. All three of them were looking at me in silence.

Rashid frowned, then seemed to regain his stance, rocking slightly on to the edges of his trainers. 'It's *OK*, ma'am,' he said to the nurse. 'I was just saying hi.' He looked from the nurse to me and raised his eyebrows.

Bertie was still frozen, unsure whether to defend himself or to play dead.

The nurse was jabbing at a bit of loose hair behind her ear. 'Well, OK – but no *touching* please, he might not like it. You have to give people their personal space here.' She paused to let this sink in, then nodded. 'Thank you.'

The three of us watched her veer out of the room.

'What the . . . ?' Rashid stared after her, shaking his head.

Bertie continued to stare forward blankly. The socks swung in his hand as he turned.

'See you later, brother,' Rashid said as he watched him walk away. He rocked on to the edges of his trainers again, his long face thoughtful. 'This place, man!' He breathed out. 'You know, I really been *thinking* about these wards. So, hear me out. People in England, yeah? They go off to Africa to help people, right? But look here! All around are people who need care, mostly Black guys, Brown guys. But off they go, off to Africa. And who are we left with?'

Later that day, Rashid was in the day area watching TV. The hand on the clock had moved to seven which beckoned the evening medication round. Rashid's name was being called.

'No thanks!' he said over his shoulder from the sofa. 'I'm feeling OK without it! I'll sleep OK, thanks!'

Silence. No one came. I could feel a hum of anxiety gnawing at me, my eyes darting from Rashid to the open door.

The minutes ticked by. *Something's wrong*, I thought, *they must have forgotten. They never let that happen.*

Then, Ray was standing over him. 'Please, Rashid,' she said. 'Reconsider. Your medication is important.'

Rashid repeated himself: 'No, thank you. I'm fine today, ma'am.'

Another nurse joined them. 'You're not *well*,' he tried to reason. 'You must take your medication, it's in your treatment plan.'

Several patients were watching covertly from where they were sitting, only their eyes shifting in their static frames.

Leon appeared out of nowhere. I didn't know he was back on our ward.

'OK – up!' Leon said to Rashid.

Rashid didn't move.

Leon lunged forward and tried to pull him to his feet. Rashid pulled his arm back vehemently.

'Hey!' he said.

'Stupid man!' Leon barked.

Rashid's mouth hung open in shock. 'What the – anyone else *hear* that?' He looked around frantically. No one answered him.

'Come to the hatch *now*,' Leon said, grabbing his arm again.

'I don't want it.' Rashid's voice was rising. 'It doesn't make me feel good!' His voice louder now. Urgent. 'It knocks me out!' He looked at the faces of the staff around him. 'Hey – hey. Are any of you *listening* to me?'

There were more staff now, and Rashid was standing up. He began to shout. 'What do you want from me? Why don't you all leave me alone? I don't trust any of you!'

Leon went to take his arm again and Rashid pushed him. 'Hey! Don't touch me! I don't know you! Get off me!'

Someone pulled their alarm. It blared through the ward, deafening. Rashid was calling out over the din: 'Help! Help!'

Our eyes locked across the room. He shouted again, shouted my name. I couldn't move. The room was collapsing. Shapes were piling on to one another. There was nothing, nothing I could do.

Nurses were running past me. The alarm throbbed. My mouth was moving, but no sound escaped. Three nurses pinned Rashid down as he tried to kick them, punch them. I saw Fuad's face behind, pained, hollow. A nurse was flicking an air bubble to the top of a syringe.

The incident was recorded in Rashid's notes. Staff described him as 'paranoid', 'suspicious' and 'aggressive'. Dr Oxley called Rashid's parents to tell them that their son was *still unwell*, that his behaviour may be symptomatic of a long-term psychotic disorder like schizophrenia, that he required further monitoring. But that they shouldn't worry. Their son was in the right place. He was in safe hands.

Fuad and I were sat outside the hospital on the kerb of the pavement. He was holding his forehead in his hands, his eyes closed. The wind had picked up around us, tearing through the scraggy bushes. Somewhere, something loose and metal was squeaking.

I watched Fuad's body rocking gently. He rolled his head towards me, his hands still taking its weight.

'Well, *fuck*,' he said.

He took a deep breath.

'I'm sorry.' His jaw looked stiff. 'I don't like to curse.'

It was the first time I'd seen Fuad truly angry. His eyes looked irritated and bloodshot.

I felt a sharp pain and looked down at my hand to find a deep half-moon indent in the skin below my knuckles where I'd been pushing my nail into the flesh. I stared at the shape, ran my finger over it. Watched it begin to fade. I didn't feel anger any more, I realized as the red line grew pinker, just a peculiar, dreamlike calm.

'So.' Fuad lifted his head up and squinted into the wind. 'Let me think about that – that *scene* – as a Black Muslim man. *Can I?*' He was almost spitting the words.

I nodded.

'What I wonder is,' he continued, 'how consultants are deciding who's psychotic, even *schizophrenic*, and who has PD if they're all saying the same stuff? Do they look at a white boy and say, Oh – he doesn't want his medication, he's making strange stuff up about secret missions, but he doesn't *really* believe it. He's just *manipulating* me. Whereas this Black guy, he doesn't want his medication either, he's been acting strange, shouting about his scary religion. He's *dangerous*. He's got schizophrenia. One's a joke, and the other is . . . is . . .' He clicked his teeth. 'One stays here, and one gets out. You see what I'm saying?'

I nodded again, feeling the weight of his words. I had noticed the number of diagnoses of psychosis or schizophrenia seemed higher with Black men and women than among white patients.

*

Decades of studies illustrate the significant disparity between the frequency of schizophrenia-spectrum diagnoses given to Black and Brown persons compared to white persons, with those with Black Caribbean or Black African heritage diagnosed at higher rates than any other group. These stigma-laden diagnoses invoke a pervasive fear in others and have lifelong consequences: an increase in punitive forced treatment and physical restraint, higher doses of medication and decreased options for psychological support, reduced career opportunities, substandard medical and social care, and increased contact with legal systems. As a result, Black and Brown patients are more likely to experience a poor outcome from treatment and to disengage from mainstream mental health services.

Recent research outlines how differences in the frequency of patients given schizophrenia-spectrum diagnoses are not due to genetic reasons – as decreed for many years – but instead occur largely as a result of the societal racism and cultural illiteracy that poisons attempts at objectivity within psychiatric diagnosis. It is acknowledged that higher rates of traumatizing stressors lead to Black and Brown individuals being more likely to experience complex distress, yet their presentation is *less* likely to be acknowledged within psychiatry as post-traumatic than for their white counterparts.

Figures show that far from improving, racial inequalities in our mental health services are widening. According to official NHS data, Black patients being restrained in mental health care has more than doubled in the past six years, widening the gap with other racial groups. Black patients are four times more likely to be restrained or held in isolation, with the numbers being injured or dying as a result of restrictive practices having risen by as much as 20 per cent in recent years.

*

Fuad was looking away into the wind again. Behind us, a bin fell over. He didn't flinch.

'That's it,' he said under his breath. 'I can't – I just *can't* – do this.'

I swallowed. The odd calmness in me knew what was coming. The outline of two feelings appeared: loss – for myself, for everyone on the ward; and gratitude – for Fuad, for everything he was, and for this gift to himself.

But what about me? Could I do this job?
'What will you do?' I asked, shaking the thought away.
'I'm going.' He was nodding, willing himself on. 'I'll go to that place, I'll go to The Garden, I will.' He turned to look at me. 'This isn't me. This isn't *me*.'

6

The Beehive

Fuad was signed off sick, and the days dragged desperately without him. I buried myself in the beehive. Today, as usual, it was a hum of activity. A crush of staff busying themselves inside its cavity. All computers were lit up: nurses scrolling through discount clothes stores, typing notes, pointing out places they wanted to holiday. There was a whirr of constant movement, keys clanking, drawers opening. Footsteps knocking back and forth as besieged nurses took turns fielding noisy requests at the door.

The cluster in the beehive was forever under attack. An unrelenting wash of sadness engulfed it from all sides, a pounding, indeterminable need that became horribly monotonous. The glass dome was a barricade from the battle. It cast those outside and those within as adversaries, fuelling an expanding distrust and hindering empathy.

Perhaps the enclosure was respite from the web of uncertainty and inarticulate demand, the daily brutality of being unable to relieve the distress of a desperate person. Nurses who were powerful, but gasping for control. Recognized, yet wholly unseen. Definite; excusing. Nurses: loaded with an indescribable weight.

There comes a point under this burden when the brain goes into shutdown. It moves past fight or flight into disassociation. Unable to take it any more, it goes offline. Overwhelmed, the emoting parts of our brain detach. The mammalian parts are activated. We move through the world disoriented, as if we no longer belong to it. What was once familiar and demarcated appears as functional reproduction stripped of meaning. A disturbing, uncanny chasm opens.

And from within this uneasy disconnect, we perceive threat. We sense our isolation in the world, the tenuity of our mind's acceptance of the reality we're trapped in. As our despondency grows, it's easier to just follow orders, to numb ourselves, to hide amid banality.

Sometimes it takes only a single second to descend into this shock. Something cuts into the unspeakable. For me it was Rashid. The magnification it brought to my own complicity and entanglement. I'd dared to connect with him, offering a normalcy and optimism I could not fulfil. To unite and then acquiesce is an unendurable loop, and to disconnect is our fragile mind's bid for survival.

'You missed all the drama again.'

Gabe was leaning against a desk, his long legs crossed.

'Oh?'

I felt myself want to sneer at him. He dug at a tooth with a fingernail, making this option even more appealing.

'Jesus got a *little* angry last night,' he said.

Colin believed he was Jesus. It was a common delusion.

So common, in fact, that it has become part of the canon of clichéd depictions of madness.

When Colin arrived, having been found climbing someone's drainpipe in a bid to preach from the roof, a nurse had nodded knowingly. 'Every ward has to have a Jesus,' she said. 'We were due one.'

I pivoted, wanting to get as far away from Gabe as I could.

'Hey!' he called. 'Where're you going? There's a meeting here now.'

I raised my hand in recognition and swerved away from the beehive door, feeling a dullness clouding me. *Always another meeting.*

Nurses started to gather near the whiteboard, turning in their chairs or propping themselves up against furniture. A nurse who looked to be in her early twenties walked in from the hallway, her eyes down. She stopped beside me, introduced herself as Andrea, and shook my hand awkwardly, before rubbing at the shaved side of her head.

'Sorry,' she said, laughing. 'I don't know *why* I do that, like I'm in a business convention or something.'

Gabe's voice was behind me, too close to my ear. '*An-drea,*' he drawled, 'what happened last night, huh? That's not what we call being a team player.'

Andrea turned away. She had a strong climber's back. 'Great – well, *sorry*,' she replied testily, not looking at him.

Gabe didn't get the hint. 'Andrea didn't want to give Jesus a tranq,' he told me, and grinned as if this were a punchline.

Andrea sat down. 'I didn't *not* want to, as I explained,' she said, still looking away from him. 'I was just ... my hand wasn't still enough.'

Gabe found another nurse's eyes and rolled his.

The nurse looked at Andrea. 'It's OK,' she offered, kindly. 'He's just kidding around.'

Andrea was silent.

'OK – hi, everyone.' Ray was standing by the patient whiteboard, a pen in her hand. 'I hope we're all feeling all right today.' She looked around the circle of faces. 'Just a few things to note. A young man called Denzel has joined us, he's in his bedroom sleeping. He was upstairs in PICU for a night, though seems stable now. But we might want to give him a temporary one-to-one, as he also has a messiah complex.'

Laughter rippled around the room.

'*Two* Jesuses?' someone interrupted.

Ray smiled. 'Yes, that is the situation.'

The conversation quickly steered from jokes to concern, as staff worried how Denzel and Colin would interact.

'Colin was crying this morning,' a nurse said. 'He's still very volatile after last night, and still very delusional. I don't think he's going to like someone moving in on his patch.'

'They might not tell each other if we don't say anything,' offered another.

'Don't put them in any groups together,' a sombre care assistant cautioned. 'They might go for each other *big time* – I've seen it before.'

After tasks were assigned and treatment updates handed over, everyone filtered out. Ray stopped me in the doorway, her hand on my elbow. 'Do you have a few minutes?'

Her face was as unreadable as usual. I felt my stomach twisting. *What was it this time?*

'Sure,' I said, not feeling it.

We waited until the last nurse had left. For the first time I'd ever experienced, the beehive was silent.

'Oh good,' she said, looking around at the swirl of chairs.

We both sat down, and Ray tilted her head thoughtfully.

'I was hoping to catch you today...'

She paused, and for a moment I wondered if she was nervous.

'Oh?'

'I can see that, well, things have been *difficult* recently,' she said softly. 'Haven't they?'

I looked at her, surprised. 'Um' was all I managed.

She looked away briskly, as if to inhibit the possibility of further emotion. 'So, I wanted to pass on,' she continued, half to the wall, 'that I see you're doing a good job.' She smiled her strange, unreadable smile. 'Honestly. Just to say, I know you're finishing with us soon, and if you'd like a job here when you graduate, I'd welcome that.'

I felt a pummel of unexpected gratitude – at her sentiment, her warmth. Warmth that was so rationed in this place, when it came it could bowl you right over. 'Thank you,' I said, feeling both honest and fraudulent, a lump pressing into my throat. Though I *was* thankful, deeply thankful, for her acknowledgement, it came with a flicker of shame at the concreteness of my other full-bodied but silent response: *No, never. I can't.*

Weeks and then months had passed, burrowing without any light; I no longer knew why I was continuing. Though I'd passed through the centre of a tunnel, I thought, and might as well continue forward, Ray's reminder of the end was welcome. I knew I only had one more rotation ahead of me: the hardest part was surely over. Could I be this person for ever? Could I, like Fuad, seek out hospitals where hope remained high, or navigate the wards, like this one, that so desperately needed staff? Was there a way to bend this doctrine, a way to be part of change? I so badly needed something, anything, to cling to.

When I left the beehive, Colin and Denzel were in the hallway talking. I watched them smiling at each other, their bodies relaxed, their posture open. I closed the door carefully behind me, as if an unexpected noise would break the spell.

'I'll *beat* you though,' Colin was saying, 'and it'll probably be painful.'

Denzel pushed out his lower lip and shrugged. 'Can't play without chips, man.'

'Well, that's true . . . true. Maybe I could get some coins, or . . . anything really could work.'

'Not the same though,' Denzel said.

'True, my brother, true.'

Two looming men from different worlds, I thought. A wealthy white man who moved back into his parents' house at forty-one after his business and relationship collapsed, and a thirty-two-year-old Black man, unable to work or leave his sick mum's home where he helped care for his disabled brother. The delusions had crept up on them slowly, with remarks to family and friends about how much they just *knew*, about everything they were *really* good at. So good, in fact, that *they* came up with the premise of that TV show, *they* painted that impressive mural. They turned down film parts, they won at high-stakes poker. They could just *feel* who was lying and who was telling the truth. They knew what the news was before anybody spoke. They were underappreciated by the world, and then exposed by it. Deployed for their power, hunted down for their existential threat. They were too important, they felt, too exceptional for how life had turned out for them.

'I'll let you win though.' Denzel shrugged again. 'I don't need your money.'

'Money *is* but a blunt tool,' Colin said, nodding. 'I agree.'

Rashid, his face resolute, steered out of his bedroom. Moving past them, he leant in shiftily. 'Watch the fuck out, Jesus,' he said, indiscriminately. 'There's a conspiracy going on in here.'

Colin and Denzel surveyed him silently as he walked away.

As Rashid passed me, he nodded in acknowledgement, his face still. I smiled, barely able to look at him as guilt gnawed into me. I wanted to shrink into the wall.

'*Life* is a conspiracy,' Colin said to Denzel, wistfully.

'He *knows*.' Denzel folded his arms across his chest and nodded. 'They all *know*.'

'Brother,' said Colin, 'I will keep you safe.'

'I trust you not to snitch,' Denzel agreed. 'I'm here to protect you.'

I watched the unfolding scene, grateful for them both. For their acceptance and grace towards each other, for being better than we'd predicted. Even if it was only temporary, they were surpassing this place.

Then, as quickly as it came, my moment of contentedness dissipated, and something uncomfortable washed over me, a presence at my side. Looming. I turned to see a large man wearing only socks and shorts standing inches away. The skin on his body was glossed with sweat, his eyes still bloodshot from the irritant spray the police had used on him. I recognized him as one of the men admitted last night, and smiled.

His large body rotated towards me. 'You fucking smiling *whore*,' he growled. 'I can make demons come out of my legs.'

'Hey!' Leon was striding briskly towards us. 'Enough of that! You'll go to PICU if anything else like that comes out of your mouth.'

I was frozen, a thick fog clouding the danger. I heard myself mumble a thank you to Leon as he led the man away. My body shrunken, tiny. I wanted to be picked up and taken far away from here.

Who did I think I *was*? Calmly strolling around, believing everything would be fine. How different was I from the two Jesuses? Had I inflated my own self-importance just to survive psychologically in here? Perhaps my naive sense of safety relied on staff like Leon and Gabe wrestling others to the floor. The reality was that I wasn't safe, no one was. Neither patients nor staff. Yet, as a student nurse, I occupied a unique position within the psychiatric maze. My time there was finite. I had less paperwork, less pressure and responsibility. I wasn't seen as the jailer, so I could *observe*. I could ask and listen and absorb, read through years of notes, compare assessments, look for inconsistencies. I was both powerless and powerful.

I could stand back from threat because other staff ran again and again towards it. How many times had they been hurt or intimidated, asked to carry out orders they morally disagreed with? And what does that do to us, to our minds, and crucially to our empathy, so integral to effective mental health treatment?

'Do you want to come up and see the empty floor?' Andrea, the young nurse, had appeared next to me in the hall. She'd put on a tie-dye T-shirt and looked like she was going to a nineties squat rave. 'Maybe you've already been, but if you haven't . . . it's pretty creepy.'

I looked at her, still dazed. Wrestling with my discomfort at having been grateful, even momentarily, for Leon's presence.

'You all right?'

I nodded.

'Cool,' she said, looking away. 'Come with me.'

I hadn't been to the other floors of the building. The proposition was inviting, especially right then, when every surface was reflecting back at me disapprovingly.

'Thanks,' I replied. 'I could use the break.'

Andrea smiled. 'I like wandering about up there on my lunch break, for some reason. Pretty weird, I know.'

Leon was still talking to the man in socks as we passed. I thanked him again, as my hollowed-out body moved past his.

'Sure,' he nodded, his face serious.

As we closed The Door behind us, Andrea leant closer to me. 'Watch out for him,' she said. 'He was my friend's nursing mentor and he's a total *tool*. Whenever he was in a bad mood he wouldn't sign any tasks off her book, for no reason. She ended up finishing the placement without passing.'

We walked side by side up three flights of stairs while Andrea told horror stories about getting trapped in lifts. When we reached her chosen floor, it was unlit and hushed.

We walked around a wide square of hallway past closed door after closed door. Andrea seemed calmer here, her rhythm slowing.

'These rooms were meant to be therapy spaces,' she said. 'Pottery, cooking, yoga, that kind of thing. They were closed because of funding, apparently.'

I peeked through the glass windows. Many of the rooms were stripped bare; only the light bulbs remained. Other rooms had been temporarily occupied by displaced, amalgamated mental health teams from around the area. They must have been elsewhere now, trailing scattered boxes and teacups. Their team names were scrawled on bits of Blu-tacked paper fixed to the doors. You could still make out 'Art Therapy Club' and 'Creative Kitchen' beneath the cursive.

'How long have you been a nurse?' I asked Andrea.

She looked up at the ceiling for the answer. 'I graduated eight months ago, I think,' she said, beginning to walk again. 'I feel so fucking sick today though, honestly.' She closed her eyes as if reminding herself. 'But they couldn't find anyone else to cover, apparently. I begged. I've worked five twelve-hour days this week and I slept for, like, two hours last night. But that's nothing. My friend's working on PICU and she hasn't slept in two days. Everyone in this place is crazy.'

I considered this. 'I don't think I could do anything much on two hours of sleep,' I said, 'let alone work here.'

Andrea was peering through a door again, her hand cupped to her eyes. 'Do you know how many nursing positions aren't filled in this hospital?' She turned to me. '*Nineteen*. That's a whole two wards. Most people are locum or agency now like me, so . . .'

I was curious as to why Andrea, at the beginning of her nursing career, was working as an agency nurse. 'Don't you worry about a lack of security working a zero-hours contract?' I queried, unsure what I was really asking her.

She looked at me, confused. 'No,' she said, frowning. 'Why would I?'

'You don't want to be part of a team anywhere? Just to ... have a team?'

Whatever it was I wanted to know, I couldn't reach for it in my mind.

'Hey,' she said. 'The first year you're kind of naive about the whole nursing thing, right? The theory you learn in class and what you're actually seeing on the wards are so different. No one's actually *doing* all that therapeutic stuff in these places. They just prescribe enough drugs to get everyone through the day. I'd go back to uni, and we'd be learning about, like, psychological formulation – right? And I'd be thinking *yeah, yeah*, but how is this relevant? This doesn't actually *happen*.'

She fiddled with the sleeve of her top and looked around at the doors we'd stopped in front of. It was true, I thought. The two worlds informing our training infrequently corresponded, and yet we rarely spoke about it. A doublethink which appeared intrinsic to functioning within psychiatry.

'It's pointless to tell us that we can change things, and then when we start work – all new and keen – we're faced with *shit* hours, and so many *shit* staff, and the lack of good training or any supervision that's actually useful and isn't just my manager saying "You all right? Good."'

Andrea was red-faced now, her voice strained.

'Like last night,' she continued. 'We were restraining Colin on the floor as he was kicking off. And, yeah, I was shaking, and I couldn't inject the tranq. I was too shaky; I don't know why. So I gave it to Gabe and asked him to do it. He told about half the team after, and wrote me up for it! He says it's policy, but it feels personal.'

'He's a shit,' I said, surprising myself.

Andrea grinned. 'Yeah, he's a fucking prick.' She ran her palm across the shaved part of her head again. 'I *really* had to drink last night. It was bad.'

We walked in silence again. Somewhere above us a pipe reverberated.

'While I was working on this forensic ward,' Andrea continued, 'I had *one* clinical supervision in six months. One! And that was via email, not even in person! It's a joke.'

I watched my footfall, realizing I felt no surprise at anything she was saying, just solemn recognition.

Andrea kicked at something brown on the floor and it bounced off the wall.

'I think some staff are kind of traumatized,' she said. 'Maybe all of them, I don't know. And some are also lazy and shit and doing it just to have a job and all the overtime. Yeah – all the shit staff, all the paperwork and no one knowing what the fuck is actually going on. No thanks, I'm doing agency shifts so I don't have to care about any of that any more. I don't want to be any more a part of this shit show than I have to.'

*

Across the two years of my postgraduate mental health nursing training we had: one lecture on solution-focused therapy and how to use it; one lecture on general psychopharmacology, where a single argument advocating for each drug's efficacy was presented by a pharmacist who avoided side effects or contentious research; two biology lectures on psychiatric medication, one of which consisted of slides you clicked through online without the presence of a tutor; and two classes on psychological formulation. As students, we had to make a passionate case for the inclusion of clinical supervision to allow us to reflect on what we were experiencing on placement. It was eventually offered – for our group only – and promoted as 'optional'.

For most other professionals working with distressed people outside of psychiatry, weekly or fortnightly clinical supervision is fundamental. Yet, this offer is recurrently absent or infrequent for psychiatric staff. Studies show that 80 per cent of NHS trusts offer nurses between just four and eight sessions a year, with many sessions instead being managerial supervision where shift patterns and promotions are discussed. Crucially, there is a big difference between managerial supervision and clinical supervision. The latter is a space where a clinician, usually a psychotherapist, organizes frequent one-to-one sessions with a staff member to reflect, problem-solve, consider and evaluate their own actions, emotions and decisions within their care and treatment of vulnerable individuals. Research shows it makes care significantly safer and more effective for patients, as well as reducing stress and burn-out and increasing job satisfaction for staff.

*

Back on the empty third floor, Dr McCulloch was waving at Andrea and me from the other end of the hall, a string of colourful beads bouncing about her neck as always. She walked towards us with a wide smile.

'We meet again,' she said, 'in the corridors of madness.'

Andrea greeted her like an old friend.

'I've carved out a little private think-space up here,' the doctor said. 'Might sneak in a bed.' She laughed. 'Going down?'

Andrea's break was over and she raced ahead of us, the sound of her shoes slapping on the linoleum fading.

Dr McCulloch repositioned her glasses on her head. 'To tell you the truth, I'm steering well clear of a certain someone or I'll blow my top.'

'Right,' I said, a rollcall of names flitting through my mind.

'But listen,' she said, starting to walk. 'I want you to understand that this team isn't at its best, as you can *definitely* see. But it really isn't as bad as some. There's a ward in a different hospital – I'm not going to say it out loud here – but the staff there, you just wouldn't believe it. *So* terrible. The reports they write are a joke, it's shocking. I'm embarrassed to send patients to them. I remember when I first saw what was going on behind some of these closed doors I thought, *My God, I hope I never get mentally ill.*' She looked at me. 'Are you having lunch?'

We reached the ground floor and turned into the small snack bar branching off the main reception area. Dr McCulloch bought a KitKat, which she slipped into her shirt's breast pocket, and a tuna roll. We sat down at a wobbly metal table in an empty corner, where she spoke between mouthfuls.

'How're you finding your training?' she asked. 'Is it what you expected?'

'Ah,' I said. 'Well . . .' I looked her in the eye. Perhaps I was past being careful. My internal response to Ray's offer had surely cemented something: I didn't want this job, so did I have anything left to prove? 'It's not . . . great,' I said, feeling instantly lighter for the admission. 'I'm honestly not sure I can do this.'

'Hmm,' she said, chewing. '*Yes*. I can understand that. I can't say I've seen you walking around with a particularly buoyant expression.' She laughed. 'But honestly, when I was training I couldn't find any role models in the field. I thought, do I really want to be doing this? It's the cliché, of course – perhaps you've heard, but it's quite accurate. A lot of doctors get into psychiatry because they're rubbish at everything else, and the minority because they have a special interest or skill.'

'Is that really true?' I replied, having come across that particular insult.

She laughed again. 'See, everyone's heard it.'

I paused. 'I have, I'm afraid. I just didn't know if it was based on fact.'

'Oh,' she said, shaking her head. 'I don't enjoy speaking ill of my profession, but that's certainly something I've seen along the way. I almost quit before I had a placement with a psychiatrist working with children and adolescents. He was the first person I'd ever seen ask, "Do you think a diagnosis would be *helpful* for this child?" He taught me the value of trying to treat with as little medication as possible. Though the other options have been reducing for aeons now, so that's limited how much choice we have in the matter.'

She looked sad for a moment.

'Anyhow,' she said, standing up. 'Shall we get back to the alternate cosmos?' She launched the remainder of her roll into the bin. 'Let's go.'

As we walked back to the ward, Dr McCulloch twisted her mouth in thought. 'Mmm,' she said. 'Apologies, I shouldn't *really* be telling you all my speculations, but ... Psychiatry – it's not very scientific, though perhaps, I don't know.' She paused, her expression tentative. 'Perhaps we haven't got anything better? I'd like to know if we did.'

'Fuad!' I called.

Fuad was at the ward door, his key card in his hand. He turned towards us, his face looked smoother and fuller than when I'd last seen it.

'You're back!'

'I was just getting the strength to go in,' he said, warmly. 'I've basically been asleep all week.'

We stopped next to him.

'You been all right, love?' Dr McCulloch put her hand on his forearm.

Fuad made a noise and rocked his head back. 'Not really!' he said, kindly. 'But thank you for asking. I appreciate it.'

Ray was waving at us from behind the glass. I was reminded, then, of my first day, standing here at this door, alone: petrified, excited, proud. And now here I was again, metamorphosed, those embryonic sentiments alien to me.

We walked in together.

'I worried I would miss you,' Fuad said as the door closed behind us. 'I really thought I was going to need to take long-term sick leave. But hey.' He grinned. He looked fresher than I'd ever seen him look. 'I applied for another job, so . . . Maybe things are looking up.'

Back in the beehive, Fuad and I took a computer each. It was lunchtime and quieter than usual, but the hum of activity remained.

Opposite, I was aware of a familiar woman on a computer, a long plait of hair running down her back. Nia. I'd watched her coming and going all week, waiting for the chance to introduce myself. I'd been told she was a peer support worker – a person with 'lived experience' of using mental health services who now visited wards and community teams befriending patients, organizing activities and giving general advice. I'd been drawn to her immediately; she appeared warm and diligent. Her manner felt effortless, like someone who with every muscle of her body just knew how to be.

I was wondering how to interrupt her when a nurse's voice cut through the room.

'*Look*,' she said into the phone, her words pregnant with irritation, 'you *need* to take your depot because you'll relapse! And when you relapse I won't be here to help you because you will have done it to *yourself*.' She paused. 'Maybe that *is* what you think of me, or maybe it's just part of your illness.'

Nia seemed to freeze, her fingers hovering above the keyboard. She must have felt me watching, as her eyes met mine. She held my gaze. I realized then what it was I'd been struggling to put my finger on all week: how everything felt unusual, muted, when Nia was in the beehive. Staff spoke differently when she was there. They were more careful with their words on the phone, their voices gentler, the asides about patients ceased. Nia was an interloper. She compromised the safety of the hive, her presence blurring the partition it created, conjuring an unfavourable reflection.

The nurse put the phone down with a drawn-out breath. '*Shit,*' she said to someone next to her. 'It's the same thing over and over with some of these patients. Some of them just need to be talked to like wayward fourteen-year-olds, you know? And some of them really do just need to stay locked up. You know what I mean?'

When in the beehive, I would often scribble down what staff said over the phone or to each other. It felt like the only way I could process what was happening – recording it, staring at it, turning it over in my mind. Later, I'd press staff to elaborate on their declarations and find they'd stumble over themselves, contradicting, manoeuvring and defending a personalized, patchwork theory about mental health in which they appeared to believe entirely, despite little research I could find. With some staff my questions were a palpable irritant, and to avoid outright hostility I'd pepper them with praise or feign complete ignorance.

One nurse (I'd written) *tells me there are 'three categories' within a human brain, one being 'behaviour', another 'emotions' and the third 'mental illness'. They are entirely separate but linked together within a 'pyramid' of chemicals.* Another told me that *mental illness 'distorts the real underlying personality through chemical imbalances that can be corrected with medication'*, despite this now being widely debunked. Another explained that *'mentally ill brains are different physiologically from well brains*' and, though nothing has so far been discovered, *'we'll soon be able to see this on a brain scan'*.

Nia was still looking at me; we seemed to sense something in each other. She stood up.

'Hi,' she said, loudly. 'Do you want to take ten minutes?' She gathered her notebooks from the desk and held them to her chest. 'I'll tell you about my groups.'

We walked outside to a square of benches known as the community garden near the back of the building, cornered by raised beds with dormant wild strawberries.

'I hope you don't mind me grabbing you like that . . .' Nia had the ability to look both staunch and kind as she spoke. 'The thing is, I have to fight *constantly* here, and I'm tired. Really tired. And you seem, I don't know, sort of an outsider.'

I let this sink in. It stirred within me, awakened something.

I asked her about being a peer support worker and she breathed out, long and loud.

'Well, I'm always explaining why what I do here is necessary. I don't feel like other staff see it as a real job. It's incredibly patronizing.' Nia looked around the courtyard, her expression troubled. 'I've had a few diagnoses in my time. I used to be on an antipsychotic. When I felt stable – it'd been long enough – I stopped taking it. Then, quickly, I started to feel pretty physically and mentally unwell. I told my GP this, and he said, "That's because you're relapsing and you need to be on medication for life." And, you know, I just *knew* he was wrong. I don't know why. It just felt different.'

I nodded, enamoured. My mind flicking through all the times I'd taken a doctor's words as gospel.

'How did you know?' I asked.

'Well,' she replied, twisting an earring, 'I did loads of research and found out about psychiatric drug withdrawal – they call it *discontinuation syndrome*, to try and make you forget that these things they put us on are *drugs*, you know? I realized I wasn't relapsing at all. My body was just trying to cope with the sudden change in what I was putting into it. So, I went back to my GP, and amazingly he listened to me. He didn't know about it, most doctors still don't. They still say psychiatric drugs are not addictive, that withdrawal is mild if not non-existent. And the more I've spoken to doctors about it, the more it seemed like actually they don't *want* to know about withdrawal, they'd rather continue parroting how easy they are to come off than face any responsibility.'

'What do you mean?' I asked, feeling myself willing her on from beneath my despondency.

'Well, I mean, things like – I was running a group here with patients, and I showed a video I'd found really inspirational about two women who'd fully recovered from schizophrenia and no longer took meds. They'd found other ways to cope, and made it through withdrawal. So, I showed this video to patients, and I was actually told off by staff. Given a stern warning. They said it was irresponsible to encourage people to come off medication.'

Nia's eyes filled with tears. She looked away.

'That *wasn't* what I was doing,' she said. 'I was trying to . . . give them some *hope*.'

Hope. That's what it was. That's what was missing. I – this whole ward – so desperately, urgently, needed hope.

'Apparently I'm not toeing the party line,' Nia continued.

'But I *know* what it's like to recover. I *know* how much better I feel now I'm med free. I'm not stupid, I get that it's not possible for everyone. I just think people should be able to make their own informed decisions.'

She took a deep breath as if exhausted by the force of her words. We watched a man in a hoodie perch on the end of a bench and start rolling a cigarette.

'Do you like working here?' she asked me. 'Being in this place? You can be honest.'

I bit at my bottom lip – another incisive, direct question forcing me to face my tangled emotions. But this time I felt clear as a bell.

'I . . .' I paused, watching Nia's eyes widen as she waited for me to continue. 'No,' I said. 'No. To be honest, I feel a bit like I'm falling apart.'

Nia's eyes welled again. She looked down. 'I think I'd worry you were a robot if you weren't feeling that way.'

A panicked feeling took me by surprise. I suddenly realized I'd been hoping Nia might be the one to lift me up, show me it could all be OK. But maybe we were going down together after all, maybe it was unmanageable – she wasn't going to keep me afloat, and it was unfair to ask that of her.

'But,' she said, turning to me, her cheeks flushing with colour, 'you should come to the talk tonight.' She smiled. A wide, genuine smile. 'Nothing builds hope like a room full of people who think like you.'

I looked up at her. A dappled sunlight was falling across the side of her face.

'What talk?'

*

Nia, I learnt, was part of an interconnected 'psychiatric survivor movement', a many-pronged network encompassing patients referring to themselves as 'survivors' as well as 'critical' staff – including nurses, psychiatrists and psychologists – together with academics and journalists who all take issue with our current approach to mental health treatment. This international movement critiques the foundations and practices of psychiatry, demands more education around psychiatric medication, champions grass-roots activism, promotes alternative treatment and sets up training institutions. It tackles our textbooks and psychiatric curriculums, runs twenty-four-hour support facilities without forced detention or medication, discusses alternative frameworks of mental distress that avoid medical diagnostic categories, promotes non-drug or reduced-drug treatment, sounds the horn for decolonizing global mental health services, and confronts racism.

It was almost too much to learn at once, and after Nia left to join a meeting I stumbled back into the beehive, my mind fizzing.

That was the moment, just in time, when a new world opened up. I was ignited, hope bursting in a surge of colour. Amid all the disorder there was something to cling to; there was a way to survive. There were people within this system trying to make things better.

7

The Clozapine Clinic

I COULD COUNT THE REMAINING months on one hand, when my rotation into the community was arranged. Ray told me I would work within the clinics and teams there for two days of every week until I finished my training. I hadn't had enough exposure to depot injections yet, she said, and being out in the community would provide more opportunities to do this. She was right, though it wasn't a plan I welcomed. But this task had to be signed off, she reminded me buoyantly, and the clock was ticking for my completion.

*

Community psychiatric care is multifaceted. It exists to keep people out of hospital with the aim of addressing a patient's condition holistically. Crisis (or Home Treatment) Teams will work with patients in their home who are in acute need of support but not deemed unwell or unsafe enough to be in hospital. They may have been discharged from hospital or A&E recently and require follow-up, or been referred by their

GP. The team is meant to assess their needs comprehensively administer their medication, support them both psychologically and socially, and plan and implement their care. Yet, most of the patients I spoke to told me their experiences with these teams largely consisted of staff entering their homes and coercing or enforcing medication regimes, which appeared to be the only measurable mark of their accountability.

Other teams are more specialized, such as the Early Intervention Team, who work solely with people having psychotic experiences, again those not deemed too risky or unsafe to remain at home. Or there is the Community Treatment Team, who work with long-term patients thought to need ongoing support or monitoring. The Community Treatment Teams are for patients who either accept or are forced to accept their need for ongoing treatment. These patients are painfully referred to as 'chronic' or 'revolving door', and it's within the team's buildings that they pool away from the rest of the world, like the existential residue of our collective unconscious.

The Community Treatment Team is also the home of the clozapine clinic – the outside world's replica of the treatment room on the ward.

*

The community hospital I was placed in was, helpfully, only next door to the ward. When I arrived, it was arranged that I spend my first day with Tina, a nurse with an army-style crew cut. Tina told me she would acquaint me with the clinic – her face lighting up as she uttered its name – as we stood sheltering from the rain under the hospital entryway. She was close to finishing her cigarette when another nurse walked past and bumped her arm. Tina laughed, her cheeks flushing, and pulled another cigarette from the packet in her hand.

'I'm the cigarette dispenser.' She smiled at me in explanation, as she handed it to the nurse.

'You look after me well!' the nurse said, returning the smile.

Tina's eyes followed the nurse silently as the door closed behind her. She cleared her throat and gazed at something invisible to me, stubbing her cigarette out on a bin and folding it over and over on itself with ritualistic precision.

'Right,' she said, clapping her hands as if to wake herself. 'Done.'

I followed Tina into the building and through the reception area, almost identical to my ward next door. Yet, in comparison to that reception which was always empty, the entry point to the community teams felt like a train station in rush hour. I glanced around as I walked, weaving through bodies. A woman wearing what looked like four jumpers layered on top of each other was draping a large blanket over several chairs, and a round man in a beret and wellies was standing legs akimbo as if riding a surfboard in the middle of the room. Two women, one knitting and one shouting conversationally at the other, sat in a corner, while in front of them a man in a denim jacket was instructing the receptionist to 'CHECK AGAIN – CHECK IT', one finger stabbing at the top of the desk.

Despite the commotion, the atmosphere felt different from the sparky volatility of the ward. There was something indescribable hanging in the air, weighty and torpid.

Tina and I stopped some way down the hallway in front of a white door. She unlocked it and pushed into a windowless room. A familiar space: all-white, wipeable daybed, a square fridge, barely room for two people to stand. The clozapine clinic was also where depot injections were given, yet the eponymous drug took so much extra time to manage that it had the accolade of ownership.

Clozapine is the most expensive antipsychotic medication available and is therefore often referred to as a 'last resort drug', meant to be given only when all other antipsychotics have been tried and have 'failed'. Its laborious management is due to its severe and potentially fatal effects, which have to be monitored fortnightly. As a result, Tina told me, much of her time is taken up by blood tests which check for a reduction in white blood cells, and completing the corresponding paperwork. She also monitored for the drug's other very common, and very serious, side effects – 'very common' being clinical terminology for side effects occurring in more than one in ten users. These included diabetes, vast weight gain, tremors, urinary incontinence, colon issues and constipation, dizziness, hypersalivation (constant drooling), extreme drowsiness, tachycardia (rapid heartbeat) and high blood pressure.

In fact, with clozapine, studies show that between 68 and 89 per cent of patients experience at least one major side effect. However, it is the more dangerous and lesser-known side effects that can't easily be monitored. New studies now prove that clozapine can cause heart failure and pneumonia, with reports from the World Health Organization showing fatal outcomes in 22,596 patients worldwide, and 6,567 deaths caused directly by clozapine in the UK. As a result, some researchers are calling clozapine the third most lethal drug in the world after oxycodone and fentanyl. Despite this, clozapine is still forced on patients under treatment orders and given without proper warning or information regarding its risk.

*

I watched quietly as Tina worked throughout the morning, wondering at the uniformly impassive and distant manner of each patient who came in. Their faces invariably sported a sickly pallor, dark circles beneath their eyes, with their stomachs protruding spherically – a common physique for anyone on high doses of antipsychotics.

With some patients, Tina was silent except for running through the side effect checklist. With others she made much more of asking about their family or home, and I would notice an echo of surprise pass over their faces as they looked from me to Tina disconcertedly. Their answers were mostly guarded but polite, though when occasionally someone began to elaborate, their answers funnelling down past pleasantries towards the murkier depths of human concern, Tina cut them short and offered up a weather report.

Despite almost all the patients taking clozapine professing to having several of the serious side effects, Tina ran through the checklist at pace, often not recording the answer they'd given. I watched her do this several times, trying to decide on a polite way to interject. After one patient left the room, I turned to her.

'Where does that information go?' I asked.

'Oh ...' Tina thought for a moment. 'General patient monitoring – back up to the psychiatrists. And data for research studies.'

I had hoped she wasn't going to say that. I'd been reading about the problems with flawed psychiatric drug research on the websites Nia had sent me. And now here I was, watching data collection fail.

'Ah, right,' I began tentatively. 'So, what happens to the people who have a lot of side effects? Do we think about alternatives?'

Tina considered this briefly. 'No, not really,' she said. 'This medication just has side effects.'

After a cigarette break, where Tina spoke at me about her previous years training in accountancy – a surprising deviation of interest – we returned to the clinic. A short, chaotic line had formed outside.

Perhaps sensing my need for persuasion, Tina selected a few patients to ask directly about their experience of clozapine. Her first interviewee looked pleased to be chosen.

'It's nice to meet Tina's students,' the man said. 'Tina's the *best* woman with a needle here, you don't feel a thing.'

Tina smiled broadly. 'Ah,' she said, 'go on ...'

'Not a thing,' the man said again.

'Have I *ever* hurt you during a blood test?' she followed up. 'What would you give me out of ten?'

The interviewee mirrored her smile, his eyes blank, and nodded a little too vigorously. 'Ten!' he exclaimed.

Tina beamed. I could feel my shoulders tensing.

'*Good*,' Tina said. 'And what about clozapine – it's a good medicine, isn't it?'

The man looked at me. 'I've been on it about ten years,' he proclaimed, as if he was heading up a speech. 'My doctor told me I'm *lucky to have it* – that it's a *great new medication*.'

Tina nodded and patted the man on his shoulder. 'Thank you,' she said. 'You're all good to go.'

The man turned towards the door and then stopped. He looked back at Tina.

'My cigarette?' he said.

Tina laughed thinly, handing him one from the packet in her shirt pocket.

'Every time . . .' she told me as he closed the door. 'It's a treat for him.'

After an hour as a spectator, I offered to take over recording side effects, much to Tina's relief.

'Bloody boring endless admin,' she said. 'Fill your boots.'

A man with pock-marked skin came in and slumped on the bed. He rolled up his sleeve silently. I waited to see if he would be one of Tina's chosen few, but she barely looked at him as she tapped at the vein in the crux of his arm. Curious as to why she avoided engagement, I decided to take things into my own hands.

'What does clozapine do for you?' I asked before I'd had time to stop myself.

I felt Tina's body stiffen. She turned to me.

'Do you feel it's helpful?' I continued, ignoring her.

The man rolled his eyes up in his still face. They rolled down again. 'I don't know,' he said.

Tina pinched her lips together. She turned back to the arm and ran her finger along the plump vein again, pushing the glinting needle through his skin in one short, sharp movement. The man flinched.

'But it's the best medication you've been on, right?' Tina said to the arm.

The man shrugged his other arm. 'I guess so.'

'Do you have many side effects?' I persisted, feeling Tina's bulk at my side. The room seemed smaller than it had been only seconds before.

The man eyed Tina suspiciously, before looking back at me. 'Yeah, some,' he drawled. 'You actually wanna hear? OK. I sleep *all* the time. I'm tired *all* the time. I can't make myself do anything much.'

Tina was peeling back the surgical gloves, pushing them into the medical waste. She turned abruptly and busied herself on the computer.

'That's not so bad though,' she said to the screen.

The man looked away, discouraged. 'I have pains in my arms too,' he offered. 'In my shoulder joints – it's weird.' He crossed his arms and squeezed them with his hands.

Tina spun on her heel, her face knotted. 'That's *not* from the medication, it would be the *first time* I've seen it.'

The conversation halted, and I managed a few rushed, reconciliatory words. The man gathered his coat and left.

Tina and I stood side by side. The fridge hummed.

'I'm going for a cigarette,' she said.

Alone in the room, the strip-light flickered above me. I was staring at the pile of unused needles on the bed when a short, punchy knock on the door made me jump. Before I could open it, a woman's puffy face peered around the door.

'Can I come in yet?' she asked.

The woman, in her late thirties, told me she was new to clozapine, only having started some four months previously. 'It's fine at the moment, I think,' she said. 'But I don't know – nothing actually ever gets rid of the voices. My partner shouts at them sometimes, and they retreat. But nothing else works. I'm not sure what the clozapine is actually doing. I guess I feel pretty sleepy now, kind of out of it a lot of the time. But I feel I have to sort of . . . *say* it's helping, so then the doctor's happy with me.' She paused. 'That sounds crazy, I don't know how to explain it.'

Tina returned from her smoke, and after a few curt pleasantries and a vial full of blood, the woman left. For a few seconds, we stood in silence.

To my relief, a man in sunglasses barrelled in, the door swinging wide.

'Hey,' Tina said sharply, 'be gentle! There's expensive medication in here.'

The man ignored her, his arms swinging wildly. 'Let's get this over with quickly then.' He rolled up his sleeve and sat heavily on the daybed.

Tina said nothing, her movements hurried.

The man looked at me over the top of his shades. 'Hello,' he said.

I watched for a few seconds, then, feeling mutinous, seized the opportunity. 'How are you finding clozapine? Do you have any side effects?'

The man pulled off his sunglasses and stared. 'What's the

point of me telling you people the side effects I have?' His voice bristled with anger. 'Yes, I have them *all*. I have loads. It makes me feel like *shit*. But when I tell you people this, all you do is give me more pills.'

Tina did a little barking laugh. 'Come now,' she said, a little too loudly. 'We're *good* people.'

'Well,' the man said, 'some of you are good and some of you are bad.'

The air in the room felt close. I could feel my heart hammering.

'But,' I said, 'do you also find it . . . helpful in some way?'

The man shot me a penetrating look. 'No, not really,' he said. 'But they *make* me take it. So I've got no choice, have I?'

The blood was drawn, and the man left.

'It's lunch,' Tina announced, opening the door for me to leave.

When we returned half an hour later Tina was talkative and smiling again. She told me about her many years as a nurse and recent move to this Community Treatment Team.

'Oh, I've worked on *every* type of ward,' she said. 'I don't mind wards. Except eating disorders, I hate those places. The patients are difficult. They have bad personalities; they lie all the time. Sorry to say it, but they're manipulative – they aren't nice people. I don't know if it's the illness that gives them bad personalities or their bad personalities that give them the illness.'

I tried to relax my facial muscles. 'Oh . . . and, and now you're in the community.'

'Yeah. But I don't do home visits. Most staff do, but I figure

I work hard to get my patients a Freedom Pass, so they can come and see *me* if they like. I don't have time, I've got things to do in the clinic.'

I nodded. Having been told that community nursing was all about home visits, I was unsure how to respond.

'Plus,' she said, 'it's so boring asking the same questions over and over and getting identical answers. The clinic is practical, it's useful. And since I have the most knowledge of medication and I'm the best at depots, all the nurses ask me to do theirs.'

I looked down at my hand to find myself gripping the pen like a staff. I thought of the needle I'd plunged countless times into something inanimate, hoping it would never become a reality. It was one of the things we *did* learn at university, alongside health care policy and writing care plans, how to restrain someone physically or resuscitate them, and how to wash our hands. We certainly had plenty of practice with intramuscular injections. We injected oranges, and then fake plastic bums. We learnt about subcutaneous and cutaneous layers of tissue, about how to avoid the sciatic nerve by targeting the upper outer quadrant.

Tranquillizers like lorazepam were thin, watery substances – a quick flick of the thumb. Antipsychotics were gluey and sluggish, the fluid slow to draw from the bottle, and slow to discharge safely into a body. You had to be measured, steady. You also had to be ready for movement, for the injection not to be welcomed by the patient.

I remembered discarding a syringe on the table in class and running my thumb over the cool, pocked skin of the fruit. It felt like the corpse of a person whose raw, sunburnt flesh had hardened into hide.

I recalled Alex simply stabbing at his. 'How is this *helpful*?' he said. 'It's nothing like an actual human.'

'Thank God,' I said.

Alex frowned. 'You haven't done it yet, have you?'

We were only four months into our placements by then, and I hadn't gone anywhere near a depot.

'You *have*?' I said, surprised.

'Sure,' he said, putting his orange down. 'I figure we're going to have to, sooner or later, so I want to be really good at it so I hurt people as little as possible.'

There was no way I could avoid giving a depot for the entire course, but I had pushed it from my mind. As ever, Alex's practical matter-of-factness caught me off guard, making me feel naive and inept.

'I just . . .' I began. 'Maybe I need the person to tell me they want it, that it helps them. I don't think I can do it if the medication is being forced on them.'

I stared at Alex's syringe, poking out of his orange like an abstract art project.

'I get you,' he said, gently. 'But we also have to pass this course to be able to change anything. There are some shitty hoops we just have to jump through.'

I was irritated, then, by the frankness of his words. But I knew he was right.

'Didn't you say we had to take down capitalism before anything could change?' I said spikily, perhaps wanting to puncture the calm confidence that was making me feel so unsteady.

He grinned and shook his head. 'That's not what I *meant*,' he answered. 'You can't look at it like that. Sure, that's the end goal, but in the meantime we just have to do everything we can – small steps. It's an unending fight we're in, but it's still worth it.'

I was desperate to change the subject before Tina asked the question I was dreading about my depot experience. 'You do have patients you key-work, right?' I asked her. 'Patients under your care – to monitor?'

'Oh yeah, I do that too – I have thirty-three,' Tina answered proudly. 'But average time we see people is once a month, for maybe half an hour or something. So, I see them in the clinic. Actually, one is coming in today so you can meet him later.'

Ian sat stiffly in a chair, one wandering eye flitting about the room, the other looking coolly at Tina. His lank, grey hair rested on his bony shoulders. Tina introduced me, then opened her arms wide like a conductor.

'Firstly,' she pronounced, 'I'd like to congratulate you on your appearance – much less scruffy.'

Ian mumbled a thank you.

'But you still smell of cat. I heard your flat is a mess and smells like cat poo. What's happening there?'

Ian was silent.

'Well,' Tina continued, 'we'll have to think if a cat is the best idea for you. You need to look after a cat, or it gets sick.'

Ian mumbled something, and Tina looked at me with raised eyebrows.

'*So*, how were your travels?' She folded her arms, her cigarettes pushing out of her shirt pocket.

I caught my breath, feeling an opening to change the tone of conversation.

'Where did you go?' I said, willing him to elaborate.

Ian brightened. 'The Ffestiniog and Welsh Highland Railway – it's a wonderful trainline.'

Tina chuckled. 'He likes trains,' she said, as if Ian was elsewhere. 'He has a lot of model trains in his house too, right, Ian?'

'What did you—' I began, but Tina leant between us.

'Ian,' she interrupted, 'do you remember why you were first put in hospital?'

I turned to her, unable to hide my bewildered expression. Ian was quiet, both his eyes elsewhere now.

'I don't know,' he said in a low voice. 'My mother put me there.'

Tina smiled. 'Yeah, it was a long time ago. Hard to remember that sort of thing. Also, I forgot to ask last time I saw you, why don't you see your sister? Because you should. On our files it says that you have *no one*, and you should have some family. What if you get sick? Anyone can get sick. You should contact her – why haven't you? It's a good idea.'

Ian's upper body appeared to have folded in on itself, his spine protruding as if to ward off this barrage of criticism. 'I don't know,' he murmured.

Disoriented, I made a few rushed comments about the difficulties of keeping in touch with family. Then there was silence.

'Please tell me the name of the journey again,' I said, feeling desperate. 'I'd like to look into it.'

Ian lifted his head, a glimmer of pleasure flitting across his face. 'The Ffestiniog and Welsh Highland Railway – it's wonderful,' he said again.

Tina checked her watch and pushed at her cigarette packet.

'Anything else you want to say to me before we end?' she said.

I left the room just after Ian and caught him in the hallway.

'I'll look that railway up,' I said. 'Thanks for the recommendation.'

Ian's face looked taut and red, his cheeks hollowed out. It was as if the anger he'd repressed in the room was now surging out of his body.

'This *bourgeois nonsense*,' he growled, walking at pace towards the door. 'Interfering with my *presentation*. I'm a free man, you know? I do and dress as I please. It's none of her fucking business to tell me how to dress. Self-care is not my fucking problem, nor is mental health. My fucking problem is *benefits*.'

I nodded, trying to keep up with him. 'I ... sorry' was all I managed.

Ian was out the door and into the world again, muttering to himself.

Later, I read Ian's care plan. As with most plans I'd seen, it was largely written from the patient's perspective by the staff. *I take my medication*, Tina had written, *to support me to remain mentally well with the aim of maintaining independence in my own home and helping me manage my illness. I will see my care coordinator to get the opportunity to express my feelings in a non-judgemental medium, to share any concerns I have, and to explore ways of coping more healthily with arising emotional issues.*

*

I avoided Tina for the rest of the afternoon, busying myself with reading client files in the large open-plan office. By the evening, I noticed staff were moving around slower, talking in hushed voices, sighing. I asked a passing nurse if something had happened. She nodded.

'A patient killed himself,' she said. 'A young man. Twenty-two.'

We exchanged sympathies. I moved over to Tina's corner and passed on my condolences. She looked up from her computer with a surprised expression.

'Oh, he wasn't *mine*,' she replied, continuing to type, then stopping to stare ahead thoughtfully. 'It's always the young men. Sad.'

She shook her head.

'That's terrible.' I sat down at the end of her desk and watched her sip her coffee.

'Back when I was working on an Acute Ward,' she said, 'oh, years ago now, there was a boy I used to spend a lot of time with. I'd sit with him, help him with his uni work, go out in the garden for a cigarette and coffee together. Just chat.' Her features seemed softer as she spoke, her eyes unfocused. 'Then one day I wasn't there, I was on some training or something. He slit his wrists.'

Tina paused and ran her fingers across her mouth in thought.

'I left after that, I couldn't go back. I kept thinking, if I'd *been there* it wouldn't have happened. And then I was scrutinized by the coroners so much – all my notes – everything I ever did with him.'

She stood up, stayed standing. Then sat down again.

'I've actually...' She paused again. 'I've had that happen three more times since. Young men killing themselves. But since the first time I make sure I write anything and everything down. I'm always thinking, am I covered? If someone scrutinized this, would I come out OK? So I always tell students to be on their guard. Always imagine that what you're doing or writing could be looked over by a coroner. And if they did, would they say it was good enough?'

I could feel a weighty sadness tugging at me. *Was I wrong to dislike this woman so much?*

'Coroners always say my notes are excellent.' She smiled broadly. 'They say they're some of the best notes they've seen.'

'That's really... good. Important,' I found myself saying, sensing that she needed something from me. Some acknowledgement which was missing deep down within her.

Tina ran her fingers along her lips again.

'Depots require skill,' she said to herself. 'All this other stuff, all this talking, talking, does *nothing*.'

She looked over at me, her face having regained its solidity.

'How are you getting on with all the note-reading?'

'Useful,' I answered. 'Thanks for giving me the time.'

She looked pleased again. 'Sure thing. And then *you'll* be giving the depots in the next clinic.'

I felt my throat tighten.

Tina peered at me. 'You know,' she said, slowly, 'I can tell you're not that keen on medication. But let me tell you, I've been in this job a long time and when you're mentally ill, it's the only thing for you.'

She turned back to her computer.

'So,' she continued nonchalantly, 'best to brush up on the

DSM too – you need to be fluid in how to categorize each mental disease.'

Mental disease.

'The DSM is contentious,' I responded uncontrollably, my heart thumping, thinking of everything from Nia I'd been reading recently. 'I mean, it's an evolving, problematic document.' I bit my tongue, knowing I'd spoken bluntly.

Tina looked as though she had stopped breathing.

'I mean . . .' I stumbled. 'For example, homosexuality was still a mental disorder in the DSM until 1976, so we can't read it like a bible, is what I mean.'

A dark-haired nurse sitting opposite Tina looked up from his computer and readjusted his glasses. He mumbled something under his breath and Tina laughed.

'Sorry?' I said. The man looked at me.

'Maybe homosexuality *is* a mental disorder,' he said.

Tina was smiling at him, her eyes narrowed.

I looked from Tina to the other nurse in disbelief.

'You . . . don't actually think that,' I stammered, feeling my body recoil. '*Do you?*'

He shrugged, and looked away. 'Perhaps it is, and perhaps it isn't. That's all I'll say.'

The next morning, to my relief, I was back on the ward. I searched for Fuad, and found Dr McCulloch in the office instead.

'Ah hello,' she said, rotating on her chair to face me. 'Do you have a moment to come with me?'

'Sure,' I said.

She stood up. 'I think you'll find this interesting, if – well, "interesting" probably isn't the best word.'

I followed the doctor some way down the hallway towards the fire door, weaving around patients. My chest felt tight, a tension running across my shoulders. My body now so familiar with the adrenalin-fuelled preparation it needed to confront the unknown.

At the end of the corridor a dishevelled man was writhing up and down, looping about himself. As the man walked, his arms flailed erratically in front of him. I watched, engulfed by an eerie chill. What I was watching was reminiscent of something from a horror movie. The trajectory of the limbs was all wrong, the elbow contradicting the wrist as it contorted away from the fingers. His twisted head jerked forward, lips writhing away from the teeth, tongue curling boldly outwards, his eyes scrunching into walnuts. He looked as if he were a ragdoll caught in the wind of an industrial fan.

'What is . . .' I stared, unable to find the words.

'Hmm' was all the doctor said.

'Is he . . . is it Parkinson's, or . . .'

Dr McCulloch shook her head. 'No. This is tardive dyskinesia. A neurological disorder caused by long-term antipsychotic use, unfortunately.'

'What?' I turned to her, cold shock gripping me. 'Those movements are caused by the medication?'

'Mmm,' she said. 'Yes, I'm afraid so.'

'But—'

'It's irreversible too.'

'It's . . . irreversible?' I couldn't get my mouth to catch up with my whirring mind.

The man was still pacing. Thrashing through the air.

'Well, yes. Sadly. This is probably one of the worst cases I've seen. Its intensity can be reduced by stopping the medication, but it will still be there.'

Dr McCulloch fingered the glasses around her neck. I thought she looked unwell.

'Hey!'

Fuad was behind us. He stopped and followed our gaze.

The doctor ducked her head ruefully. 'I was explaining about TD,' she said to him.

'Oh yeah . . .' Fuad replied, watching the man. 'Terrible.'

This seemed insufficient to me. I could feel my face burning, my chest tight. 'But how many people taking antipsychotics does it happen to?'

They looked to each other. Dr McCulloch actually coughed.

'Yes . . . it's not good,' she replied. 'The statistics say about twenty-five per cent. But they aren't all as bad as he is, of course. Mostly it can look like shaking, or stiffness. Sometimes the mouth will move strangely.'

There was silence.

The man's limbs billowed in front of him. He hollered momentarily at the wall, a wordless sound.

'Often, if you see it's happening early on, you can catch it before it gets too bad,' the doctor continued. 'And maybe change drugs, if you can. But someone has to be watching *very closely*, so in the Community Treatment Team – as you've probably noticed – or for patients in assisted housing, you can imagine how frequently the early stages get missed.'

'But,' I tried again, unable to get my words out. 'But I've never heard patients being warned about it. I mean, I've never heard of it before.'

'Well, there's some information on the leaflets, though

you're right it doesn't tell them this, *exactly*. But you have to weigh up the benefit of how much you tell them about the medication. You don't want them to be too scared to take it at all.'

Fuad murmured something under his breath.

I felt suffocated.

'So . . . those movements, his . . . disfigured movement . . . is caused by *our drugs*?'

I spoke the last two words slowly and deliberately. I wanted our culpability to be heard. I wanted it to ring in the air.

Later, I checked the man's drug chart. He was still being injected with an antipsychotic called haloperidol, alongside another, olanzapine. Knowing these drugs had caused – were continuing to cause – this dyskinesia, and that he didn't know this, was too much to bear. I couldn't bring myself to speak to him. Probably like so many other staff, I just couldn't face him. I knew that if I stood in front of him, spoke to him, I'd be unable to continue to go in, with my nurse's watch clipped to my belt loop, my polished nursing shoes, ticking through my student task sheet. I wouldn't be able to continue past that moment: everything I was barely clinging to would have fallen away if I'd acknowledged my part in his pain. I was complicit by even knowing the clandestine decision that continued to be made daily by staff: that these contortions were better than the unknown. That perhaps his physical health was less important than his mental health. That maybe he wouldn't mind as much as a 'sane' person.

*

Psychiatric polypharmacy – the prescription of two or more psychiatric medications concurrently – is ubiquitous despite research indicating its substantial harms. These include greater frequency of significant adverse reactions, among them cognitive decline and brain damage, neurological disease, diabetes, a deterioration in general physical wellbeing and early death. In fact, studies show no or limited long-term advantages of polypharmacy over monotherapy for many people, with indications that these drugs could be causing transient symptoms to become chronic, lifelong issues.

Yet, despite all the serious risks associated with polypharmacy, there has been an exponential rise in its use within our mental health system, including in geriatric and paediatric patient populations. Studies highlight that almost 59 per cent of mental health inpatients have an inappropriate prescription, with up to 33 per cent having a potentially serious or fatal inappropriate prescription. Much of the danger appears to come from poor or infrequent medication reviews and monitoring which could allow for deprescribing, with as much as a fifth of mental health patients having not had a review in the previous twelve months.

*

The following morning I was back with Tina in the windowless clozapine clinic. An array of needles were spread on the sideboard next to a packet of surgical gloves. Every few minutes the fridge interrupted its hum to splutter desperately.

'This is Cheryl,' Tina said, gesturing to the woman sat on

the bed in front of us. 'You started clozapine two weeks ago now, right?'

Cheryl moved her round, flat face. It was colourless within a mass of tangled grey-streaked hair. 'Yeah, I guess that should be right,' she said, without inflection.

'It is,' replied Tina, checking the computer.

Cheryl was making a shape with her fingers, pressing the tips together. 'Lithium, sodium valproate,' she said, 'erm, citalopram, clozapine.' I watched her screw her face up, and then relax it again. 'Olanzapine?' She frowned.

'They stopped that one,' Tina replied.

Cheryl went back to her shape-making. 'Yes . . .'

'And you're still on the depot injection,' Tina said. 'For risperidone, which is being phased out.'

Two mood stabilizers, an antidepressant and two antipsychotics. So much medication moving within this soft body.

'Yes,' Cheryl said again.

There was a sudden clatter outside the clinic door, followed by a man calling out for Tina. *Tina!*

'Oh shit,' Tina said flatly. 'I told them not to give his umbrella back.' She turned to me. 'I'll be a few minutes.'

The door closed behind her. I looked at Cheryl, and she looked back at me with sunken, owl-like eyes.

'I wonder what he's *doing* with his umbrella,' she said, a faint smirk flitting across her face, before fizzling out like a choked flame.

I grinned back at her, trying to catch it somehow, to give it life. 'Whatever it is sounds exciting,' I said.

She paused. The fridge chortled.

'Would it help you to know my diagnosis, that sort of

thing?' she offered. 'I know you students have to write about us. You're always so busy.'

A sadness washed through me. Again, that gulf between us.

'I'm forty-nine,' she began, not waiting for an answer. 'I've been a patient since I was sixteen.' She rattled off a list of teams she'd been under like a register. 'I have hallucinations – rats, mostly, and snakes. And voices. I have three voices. I'm actually a member of the royal family, but they've disowned me now.'

'Oh?' I said, surprised by the matter-of-factness of this admission.

Cheryl sighed, as if preparing herself for my inevitable rebuttal. 'And, I want to improve my *small talk*,' she said. 'So I can fit in better.' Again, a knowing smile rose and faded.

The door pushed open.

'Sorry, sorry,' Tina said loudly. 'All sorted.' She turned to take a small glass bottle out of the fridge.

'No apologies,' Cheryl said. 'We were talking. It's nice to talk.'

'Oh good,' Tina answered, sounding genuinely grateful. 'You two should arrange some key-working meet-ups. It'll give you lots of time to talk.'

I nodded keenly at Cheryl's open face. 'Yeah, that'd be great, if . . . you wouldn't mind?' I said.

Cheryl's eyes widened. 'Yes, thank you.' She looked energized by the idea, her skin brightening. 'My twelve sessions of therapy ended last year, and I've missed the intelligent conversation.'

'Oh, great,' I said, feeling an excitement laced with nerves. It was a feeling I often got around patients who I sensed needed desperately to speak. An apprehension at the possibility of disappointing them or not being good enough, mixed with a latent hope. It was in these moments of connection with patients that I could still find it.

Tina was drawing up medication from the bottle into a syringe. 'Good stuff,' she said. 'Oh, and it won't be *me* giving you your depot today, Cheryl.'

I felt the air leave my body. No, no, *please*.

Cheryl was silent.

'Do I . . .' I didn't want to plead, but I really did. 'Am *I* . . . doing it? I haven't done it before, I mean.'

I turned to Cheryl, who looked unfazed.

'Go ahead,' she said flatly.

'Can't avoid it for ever,' Tina said, smiling at the needle in her hand. She withdrew it from the bottle and replaced the cap over the flash of silver. 'It's easy. You'll see. And Cheryl here is a *perfect patient*.'

She passed the needle to me upside down. I held it in my hand. It was light and slender – *No big deal*, I thought. *It is medication, right?* What could I really do anyway? Could I object? Would that even be the best thing for Cheryl? I thought of the nameless writhing man on the ward, whom I'd pushed to the periphery of my consciousness.

'I'm so sorry,' I said, light-headed, 'I don't want to hurt you.'

'It's fine,' Cheryl said. 'It'll be fine.'

'I'm sorry,' I said again, trying to swallow. 'I'm so sorry.'

I felt like I was grasping at something bigger than I could articulate. Bigger than I could conceive of.

Cheryl turned her face to the wall.
'Do you want me to lie down?'

Cheryl and I spoke over coffee twice a week. We'd meet at her flat, where she'd always forgotten to do something, and I'd follow her inside to wait. She excitedly introduced her cat, Mervin, every time like it was the first, and would become animated as we walked together to her favourite restaurant chain. We didn't talk about her mental health; instead we talked about books, politics, Mervin. She told me about her childhood, how she'd never felt as though she fitted in, how she was dogged by a sad, muted sensation. How she'd struggled to cry.

'My mum told me she wished she'd never had me,' she said one day, a half-finished cappuccino in her hand, foam on her upper lip.

Sometimes she spoke about the rats at the corners of her vision, other times she would stare into the air intently, eavesdropping on the cacophony in her head. But I noticed that each time she described her unusual experiences to me, her body seemed lighter, as if having taken off a heavy coat. She'd laugh at my intrigue, dumbfounded by my lack of derision or surprise.

'You don't think that's *weird*?' she'd say. 'You don't think *I'm* weird?'

Yet, each week I watched Cheryl physically deteriorate. The smell from her flat reached the doorway. Peach stones rotted on tabletops, dirty plates littered the floor. The washing basket overflowed on to the streaked carpet, her bedsheets balled up next to the litter tray mounded with faeces, the mattress naked and stained. Her energy seemed to be draining from her, her ability to move, to talk.

Now in the coffee shop there was often food down Cheryl's top. Her leg hair was long and stuck to her skin with sweat and dirt. Her thoughts, once sharp and droll, seemed to untether from her before they'd found a purchase.

I asked her about her new medication, clozapine.

Like a switch had been flicked, she repeated the language I'd heard over and over in the clozapine clinic. 'It's OK,' she said. 'Dr Evans says it's the best drug available.'

Dr Evans, whom I'd seen only fleetingly. A reedy, bustling woman moving through the reception area with a pen tucked behind her ear.

I pressed Cheryl to elaborate, trying again and again to elicit a personal response of some kind.

'I don't know,' she would say. 'Dr Evans says . . .'

'What would *you* like to change?' I tried. 'What feels helpful to *you*?'

Cheryl would shake her head. 'I'm just so tired all the time now. So . . . dazed.'

At our last coffee meet-up, Cheryl was almost mute. The clammer of conversation around us swelling in and out of attention.

'Sometimes,' she said, turning to me, 'I feel like I can't even motivate myself to speak any more, let alone do anything else.'

I leant in towards her, trying to reach something. 'If clozapine doesn't suit you, you must tell Dr Evans.'

Cheryl fingered the handle of her mug and looked away. 'I don't know,' she said. 'They tell me it will get better. They tell me I'm lucky to be on it.'

*

Back in the Community Treatment Team office, I trawled through Cheryl's notes. I learnt that she had severe tachycardia and hypertension from long-term psychiatric medication. I read nurses' entries. *She's sleeping from two a.m. to midday*, one had written, *then three p.m. until seven p.m. each day. She is very constipated*, said another, *and has had two recent falls due to feeling extremely light-headed. Cheryl is experiencing a dry cough and occasional swallowing problems*, another note read. *She has urinary incontinence at night and occasionally when standing.* One entry noted that she was rushed to hospital with a raised blood sugar level and sky-high blood pressure.

No change in mood was a frequent admission. As was *the dysphoric highs, visions and paranoia continue without improvement.* One nurse queried the benefit of clozapine, reporting that her mood might be *slightly better* but that she seemed to be *physically negatively impacted* by the drug. Though regardless of this concern she claimed to have *reassured Cheryl* that these *symptoms will ease off eventually.*

Dr Evans's entries for her once-a-month review read like she was speaking about a totally different person. *Cheryl feels better on clozapine*, she noted, *it appears to be working well for her.* She summarized Cheryl as being *generally more motivated and productive.*

A flood of confusion followed by anger rushed through me. What was going on? How did nothing make sense any more? I gathered my coat and bag, my mind darting about. *Should I speak to Ray?* But she had nothing to do with this team. *Or Tina?*

On my way out of the building, I spotted Dr Evans. She smiled fleetingly, and without thinking I was talking.

'Dr Evans, have you got a moment?'

She paused, radiating disappointment, and peered at me. One more unnecessary task in her day. I explained that I was worried about someone. She nodded and pursed her lips.

'Give me two minutes?' she asked, turning round and unlocking her office door. She slipped inside.

I hovered in the hall, waiting. It was empty now except for the receptionist, the front of the building having been locked to patients. I watched him watering a sickly-looking plant on the desk with a drinking glass. We exchanged weak smiles.

Dr Evans opened the door. She'd taken her coat off, and for a moment I felt guilty for keeping her. *How relentless her job must be*, I thought, *how thankless*. Then I thought of Cheryl – her disappearing speech, her motivation draining away in her rotting flat.

'I've got ten minutes,' she said. 'Shall we?'

I told the doctor about Cheryl's downward slide over the months I'd been seeing her, of her fading conversation, the state of her home, her diminishing self-care. I told her about her inability to speak, the constant sleeping, how she described feeling *different* somehow, *drained of life*.

I looked up. Dr Evans was smiling. Confused by her expression, my speech came to a halt. An odd feeling gripped me. The feeling that although this woman was physically present, the rest of her, somehow, was not.

She clasped her hands together and gave me a look that I

could only recognize as sympathy. '*Really?*' she said. 'I think she's got better.'

I sat still, bewildered. *Did she hear me right? Had I not made any sense? Was I . . . mistaken?*

I stammered something, and the doctor smiled again. I felt like a child being admonished.

'You see, I've been working with her for almost fifteen years,' she told me. 'She's been more dishevelled than this, oh yes. She just needs a good cleaner and a good long bath. It's not to do with this medication. No, it's the symptoms of *her illness*.' She stood up. 'She's a chronic case, I'm afraid. Chronic.'

I must have thanked her for her time. I remember dropping my bag as I stood up, fumbling at the zipper on my coat. I don't remember leaving her room.

Outside, the hallway was dark. I looked down at my hands to find they were shaking. A nurse greeted me as he walked past, flipping up the hood of his rain jacket. I followed after him, pushing open the door and staring out on to the wet road.

How was it that a doctor became this way? When had she lost her will for change, her energy to try? Her belief that she could make a difference?

When I returned to the Community Treatment Team after the weekend, a meeting had been called. There were not enough chairs and staff lingered in corners, files clasped to their chests. The head nurse's pale face bowed slightly as each new person entered the room.

A patient has died from a heart attack, he said. I looked

around at the faces in the room, trying to guess who it might be.

He went on to congratulate the strength and work ethic of the team, telling everyone they'd done the best they could. He spoke gently about the coroner reports being put together and that no one should be concerned. *These things happen*, he said.

No one spoke.

Dr Evans, her arms propped on the table, wrung her hands. She looked sullen as she reiterated his words. 'I want to reassure you,' she said, 'that there is *little evidence* that clozapine triggers heart failure.'

I felt my stomach clench, suddenly light-headed. I knew this to be untrue. There was plenty of evidence, if you looked for it. It was littered across the research I'd been ploughing through at home. Especially for people who have hypertension or tachycardia.

'We've all known Cheryl a long time,' the head nurse said. 'It's a terrible, unavoidable tragedy.'

My ears flooded with static, his voice fading away.

The rest of the meeting is drowned from my memory. I know that I left early that day, numb. Heartbroken.

When I got home, I emailed Alex and Nia.

What can we do? I pleaded desperately, shaking. *Is there anything we can do?*

Nia met me in the community garden, concern etched into her features. She listened to me talking for what felt like hours, her eyes wet with tears.

Around us, pairs of sparrows bounced about each other,

puffing out their chests with boisterous intention. Their tiny bodies seemingly weightless, as if they were levitating. Their rhythmic, insistent cheeps a warning, an urgent cry.

Write it down, Nia says to me. *Write everything down. Maybe that's all we can do. Things like this happen every day and slip by unnoticed. But we can't let these stories get lost. They just can't be lost.*

8

The Living Room

WHAT CAN WE DO WHEN we're unable to complain? When we can no longer explain? We can document. We can record as an act of evidence, as the basis for examination. We can attempt to capture the disorder of the whole so we can tease it apart, see its makings, and act.

*

'What are you writing?'

Rashid was peering over me, squinting at the notebook in my hand. I looked up at him from a table in the day area. His expression was gentle, curious.

I paused. What *was* I writing?

'Are you writing about us?'

An impulse wanted to deny it. Was I doing something wrong? Did these stories even belong to me?

'Yes,' I answered. 'I'm writing about what happens here. I'm trying not to . . . forget.'

Rashid nodded. 'Good,' he said. 'Don't get all white saviour about it though – remember you got all your best lines from me.'

I laughed, and Rashid smiled – a bashful, toothy smile.

'I will.'

He looked thoughtful for a moment. 'You know,' he said, 'it's all kinds of wrong in here. People need to know. Maybe if they knew, something would kick off.'

'Yeah,' I said. 'I hope you're right.'

Later that morning with the Community Treatment Team next door, I was ushered into another meeting in the large open-plan office where the team's manager was sat within a circle of staff. He looked exhausted. I slipped through a gap in the ring and found an empty seat.

'Morning everyone,' he began, his voice coarse. 'Some more unwelcome news, I'm afraid, that most of you knew was coming. Jill is retiring as planned, but we aren't able to replace her, unfortunately. The role is being cut.'

His deputy nodded along beside him grimly, her eyes staring vacantly ahead.

'So, right now,' he continued, 'we are faced with an impossible situation.'

I looked around the downcast faces, feeling the struggle between stoicism and sullenness dragging like tidal waters.

A nurse with a grey-bearded, approachable face shook his head. 'I can't take any more patients, I *can't*. It's just *not safe*. I only meet them once or twice a month as it is.'

'I agree,' a social worker echoed. 'If they aren't going to employ anyone to take Jill's patients, then we just have to pass them back up the chain and say, sorry, you deal with them then.'

'I already have thirty-four patients,' the bearded nurse said. 'If I take a share, then that'll mean I'm up to forty. And that will be the case for all of us, right? How are we meant to even see them monthly to talk, let alone actually do anything helpful?'

Murmurs of agreement whirred around the circle. The team manager and his deputy continued to nod mechanically.

With staff positions being cut, the expectations on those who remained to absorb their patients into their own enormous caseloads seemed deeply unfair. Dr Evans, for the first time I'd seen, appeared charged with a furious vigour as she leant forward.

'The thing *is*,' she began, 'not only do we have too many patients, we have an extensive waiting list that's continuing to grow. And as we know, the people they refer to us are the *most* complex, the *most* chronic. A great deal of them may well never be discharged. It's absolutely not safe or feasible to carry on like this.'

Perhaps this was where her energy was funnelled? The war of attrition. Her attempt to protect and care for the staff she saw as deeply threatened within an unsafe system.

Afterwards, I waited in the office, unsure where to be now that I was no longer assigned to the clinic. I had only been alone a few minutes when a man I'd noticed in the meeting wearing a waistcoat and stylish, thin-framed glasses popped his head round the door. He peered at me for a few seconds.

'I'm Aran,' he said, smiling. 'Home visit?'

I nodded, noticing his lanyard. Aran was a senior nurse.

'Yeah, that would be great. Thank you.'

Still smiling, Aran beckoned me over and I followed him outside the building. There he introduced me to a freckled, curly-haired junior doctor – Erica.

'This is a *first* assessment,' she said cautiously, fiddling with the shawl draped across her chest. 'It's not very far, we can walk – if that's OK?'

Due in part to the inadequate number of consultant psychiatrists employed in this Community Treatment Team, junior doctors – despite very limited independent experience of psychiatry – played a role in assessing and diagnosing. They arrived on rotation, and were positioned front-line to see new patients.

We triangulated on the pavement alongside the main road, Aran following silently behind.

'This is actually my first acute psychiatric assessment,' Erica said, squinting into the sun.

We stopped to cross the road, and I noticed how young she was, her skin still bruised with acne, shawl slipping off her shoulder. She tugged at it.

Thirty-five-year-old Delphi, Erica told me as we walked, had been referred to us by her GP. He'd described her behaviour as *very concerning*.

We walked past a wall of garages into an area blockaded by high-rise flats. Identifying Delphi's, we curled up a stairwell and across a yellowed, concrete walkway. Delphi's flat was on the seventh floor, and Erica and I rode up in the lift. After exiting, we waited for Aran – who'd said he needed the exercise – to appear at the top of the stairs. Some time later he surfaced looking casual and unflustered, his hands in his pockets.

The three of us gathered on a polka-dotted doormat and rang the buzzer. A couple of minutes passed before a woman in a beige headscarf opened the door tentatively. Her eyes scanned the corridor as she hurried us inside.

Delphi's flat was cluttered with shopping bags, used crockery and piles of magazines. Canvases with uplifting slogans hung on the walls. CHOOSE JOY, one declared. SMALL STEPS EVERY DAY, said another. Several rested on the brown carpet against the wall – whether they'd been taken down or were yet to be positioned was unclear. At the front of the pile was a framed, longer mantra: You Matter! Your Presence On Earth Is Sacred!'

Delphi offered tea, gesturing for us to sit at the table. She moved a pile of papers and various teacups on to the floor. Aran accepted her offer, and Erica gave him a lengthy sideways glance, which he appeared not to notice.

'I'm sorry it's such a *mess*,' Delphi said, returning from the kitchen. 'I haven't had time to do much recently.'

We shook our heads and reassured her. She put Aran's tea down.

'I forgot, actually,' Delphi continued. 'I mean, that you were coming today.'

'Don't worry,' Erica said. 'Are you OK to tell us what's been happening?'

Delphi took a long breath before beginning. She told us stories of persecution and domestic violence. We were shown text messages and emails from her ex, littered with insults and threats. She described sleeplessness, fear of men following her on buses, of being watched by secret cameras. Of panicked running through the streets and phone calls from people who knew her whereabouts. She felt desperate, she said. Alone.

'I don't know if I'm *safe*,' she whispered. 'I think they're following me – I don't know if it's him, or his brother. Or . . . other people. I don't know any more.'

Erica was nodding briskly, pressing her rounded cursive into a carefully angled notebook.

Almost an hour later the three of us took the lift down, walking past the garages in silence and finding our way back to the high street. As we weaved around pedestrians, I felt coated in the poignancy of Delphi's stories and sensed a new melancholy in the faces that passed us. Erica flipped through notes from the GP as she walked, handing them to me once she'd scanned them. They detailed a past plagued with violence. One account from Delphi's sister reiterated her narrative of coercive control.

'But something feels . . .' Erica began, scratching at a patch of red on her cheek. 'It's all a bit *much* though, you know? It's gone *somewhere else* now.'

I looked at her, noticing the shawl slip from her shoulder. 'What do you mean?' I asked.

'I'm just thinking that *maybe* this ex isn't actually still in contact with her, watching her, calling her – all that. And the thing about the secret cameras and people following her . . . Maybe now she's just paranoid. I mean, there isn't any evidence that anyone is after her *now*.'

Aran frowned, his expression unreadable. 'Hmm,' he responded.

As we reached the hospital driveway and passed back into the building, he turned to Erica. 'So, what are you going for then?'

Erica stroked her shawl, wrinkling her nose. 'I think,' she began tentatively, 'possibly . . . delusions of continued persecution . . . with potential psychosis traits? I'm not sure; I'm running it by the consultant at two-thirty.'

Her shawl slipped from her shoulder again and she pulled it up briskly, before kneading the tassels with her pale fingers. Aran breathed out weightily but said nothing.

I turned to Erica, feeling winded. 'Why are you thinking psychosis?'

Erica flushed. 'Well, it's my first assessment so I'm probably overestimating just in case. But best to cover all bases to be on the safe side. The consultant will check everything over.'

Within four days, a diagnosis of 'first episode psychosis' and a prescription for the antipsychotic quetiapine appeared in Delphi's notes. I called her at home, hoping to gather more information to counter what was happening.

Delphi told me she wasn't feeling great and hadn't started taking the medication. She claimed not to know what it was for. Baffled, I put the phone down and queried her lack of clarity with Erica.

'Oh,' she replied, sat behind a desk in the communal office, 'she's very jumpy about the word "psychosis". So I didn't want to say it's an antipsychotic *yet*,' she explained.

'Is it ethical to not tell her what she's taking?'

Erica folded her hands in her lap, her cheeks blushed slightly. 'Well, the consultant says not *entirely*, but that it's necessary under the circumstances, as she's becoming quite unwell, we feel. I have a meeting with Delphi in a few days to gently tell her more about the medication and her diagnosis. I explained her symptoms and presentation at the consultant team meeting and they agreed with my analysis.'

Several days later I caught Erica in the hall and asked her about her conversation with Delphi.

'I told her the medication is for anxiety,' she whispered.

'Oh,' I said, choosing my words carefully. 'So . . . we aren't going to give her something less powerful than an antipsychotic for *anxiety*?'

Erica looked more confident this week; her shoulders seemed squarer, her neck longer. 'No,' she replied, 'because her illness has psychotic features.'

'And those are?'

'Delusions. Persecutory delusions.'

I could feel my face reddening; I felt nauseous. 'Delusions linked to her ex?' I asked. 'Being stalked, threatened. Things that *did actually happen*?'

Erica looked away. 'Yes. But her response is abnormal in the circumstances. The consultant said that was in the past, and the level of anxiety now – the worries about cameras, the feelings of persecution – is too intense.'

I could feel my mind racing. Even if Delphi asked for her medical notes a clinician could decide, with the backing of a legal team, that some of the papers requested would make her mental health worse if she were to see them, and these could be redacted without her knowledge.

'Her response is *abnormal*?' I echoed.

'Yes.'

I watched Erica's mouth twitching. Her youthful, pocked skin looked sunburnt. There was a smudge of mascara beside her right eye.

'Right, OK.' I paused. 'And that means it's not high anxiety but psychosis?'

Erica's forehead crinkled as she pulled at the sleeve of her jumper. 'Yes.'

I pushed out of the hospital feeling irate, my heart pumping, unsure where I was headed. When I reached the road I turned left towards the community garden benches, hoping I might find Nia. I almost collided with Aran.

'Whoa!' he said loudly, still managing to look relaxed. He'd unbuttoned the top half of his waistcoat to reveal a brightly patterned T-shirt and was drinking something from a can. 'What's up?' he said, smiling wryly.

I leant against the wall and caught my breath. He watched me quietly.

Aran told me he'd been working on the Assessment and Brief Treatment Wing of this team for three years, after ten years working on wards. He said he was now an agency nurse, which he described as *survivable*. As he spoke, I noticed that he seemed – away from the building – like a bird released, his arms swinging as he talked openly and keenly, his laugh warm and chesty, a grin spread across his face.

'You wanna come on a home visit or two with just me today?' he asked. 'I'll be going in a bit.'

I was intrigued; he was so different now that he was alone. Perhaps I could ask for his thoughts on Delphi.

'Sure,' I said. 'Thanks.'
'Great,' he replied. 'Meet you back here in fifteen?'

When Aran finally came back, more than thirty-five minutes later, he had a coffee in his hand and a calm, open expression. 'You look *stressed*,' he said to me, still grinning. '*Chill*.'

Aran explained his lackadaisical approach to his nine-to-five schedule – always in late and doing his best to leave early – as being due to his having 'too many patients' and handling 'too much risk'.

As we walked together, he clarified his thoughts on his caseload. 'Look,' he began, 'no one wants to do this front-line job for the money they offer – I wouldn't do it if I wasn't agency; now I make twice as much as I would do as regular staff, which is almost liveable. There're just three of us in this team, taking all the referrals, seeing some of the worst shit each day, and we're expected to be nurses and social workers and benefits advisers all in one. We're expected to deal with some huge crisis – suicide, homicide – as well as sorting someone's hoarding, getting help with cooking, sorting their finances. It takes a million things to sort a life.'

'How do you keep doing it?' I asked, feeling genuinely at a loss. 'I mean, to keep seeing this stuff day after day, and keep coming in?'

Aran grunted and smiled. 'Ah, you gotta toughen up, girl. This job is dark! It makes no sense!'

I laughed, grateful for his joviality.

'No, but really,' I pressed. 'How do you cope?'

Aran pressed his lips together in thought. 'I drink?' he offered, chuckling. 'Nah, well . . . it's difficult to, you know, see this stuff and then shut off, that's for sure. Sometimes my friends tell me I'm sat there in the pub just smiling to myself, shaking my head. It's cos I'm thinking of some funny shit some patient said, some delusion so bizarre, so fucking weird, you can't help but laugh. You *have* to laugh, you know? Sometimes I think maybe that's how I cope with it all and cut off – I laugh. I make things funny even if they're really, really not.'

He stopped walking for a moment and looked down at the pavement. I followed his gaze to a stencilled FUCK PIGS. He chuckled again, his eyes shining.

'People are *angry*, man.' Aran shook his head. 'Understandable. So yeah, I drink! But honestly, I don't think people appreciate how hard our job is. Not that I want people clapping all the time, but – yeah. I also just stay in my lane, you know? I pick my battles. Don't get involved with other people's decisions – it breaks you down.'

I watched him throw his empty coffee cup into a bin and tuck his hands into his pockets, feeling a genuine warmth towards him. His bluntness was relieving.

'About that,' I said. 'Can I ask you honestly about Delphi?'

Aran furrowed his brow, his face serious for the first time. 'Yep, bring it.'

I paused, unsure how to articulate my thoughts, before realizing I could just go with his method – blunt. I told him my concerns about our assessment.

'Uh-huh,' he said, nodding. 'You know, I'll say this: that's what happens when you have to diagnose, and that's what psychiatrists *do*. They take your big fucking mess of a story and think, How can I make this fit on a survey? Which of these lists does this story sound most like? And you can't really argue with them as a nurse, not *those* psychs anyway. It's more hassle than it's worth. They like being God. God at the top of everything.' He laughed. 'Would you listen to me? Now *I* sound nuts!'

We passed a woman with a miniature dog on a lead. It crouched down to poo, and she yanked at it to keep moving.

I considered Aran's comments. Something new had been gnawing at me in this team which I hadn't yet articulated. Now it surfaced like a diver.

'But,' I said, 'a lot of people *want* an answer from them, from us – right? They come to us *for* a diagnosis, don't they?'

'Oh, sure,' Aran replied, 'that's what they *think* they want. I mean, no one comes in wanting a schizophrenia diagnosis, but sure, people want something they think can be treated. Right? They want the magic pill. The cure.'

'Yeah. That's true.'

'They come in wanting to be fixed,' Aran continued. 'I want *you* to tell me what to do. I want *you* to give me the answers about how to *live*, how to *survive* this shit. Do you feel that pressure as a nurse? Cos I do. I feel it all the time. But often if you just listen to them, believe them, tell them you get that it's fucking hard, that there are no quick fixes but that it's survivable, then that's all good. That's all people really want most of the time.'

We walked in silence, the warm sun on our backs. *Tell them it's survivable. All this mess, all this pain. That there's no quick fix, but it's survivable, it's meaningful.*

'Shit,' Aran said. 'These buildings look great, right? Little palaces?'

I looked up. The streets in this part of the city were beautiful.

The houses were expansive, opulent even. Four or five floors with raised columned porches and large bay windows.

'Lucky people,' I said, trying to peer through into a lower ground floor.

'Or not,' Aran said, with a mischievous smile. 'They're mostly all cut up inside into council flats. You'll get a real shock when we go in one – I did. One of my patients has one of these basement flats and it's probably the worst place I've ever seen, and that's saying something. The guy's toilet wasn't working for a bunch of time and he was shitting in bags and chucking it out the back. No wonder the guy had lost touch with reality. I would have.'

'Aran,' I said, stopping, 'I really wish you'd been on my ward; it would have been easier with you there.'

Aran laughed deeply. 'Thanks, mate. But whenever I was on a ward I wanted to move again, quick. I'd keep going from ward to ward. If I stayed too long, I'd start seeing things I don't want to see. I already lost my girlfriend, a ton of my dignity – I've been called a Black bastard, a monkey, so many times – I almost lost my job by shouting at a psych. So, yeah. I choose to step out sometimes. I pick my battles.'

'I get it,' I said, thinking of Delphi. 'I really do. I didn't think I would. I mean – I didn't used to. But I get it.'

'Sure.' Aran stopped walking and put his hands on his hips. He was still grinning. 'I just *know* you came in thinking you were a Polly do-gooder.'

We both laughed.

'A *Polly do-gooder*?'

'Sure,' he said again. 'Going in thinking it's all gonna be great. That you're gonna really change people's lives. You hadn't seen anything yet! But seriously, if I got mentally unwell, I would probably hide out in my house and not tell anyone. Or I'd leave the country – I'd be gone.'

I nodded.

'I mean,' he continued, 'I went to the GP with a migraine about a year ago. He wasn't even listening to me as I was telling him about it. He started asking me about stress, kept talking over me. Then he said, "I'm going to give you a prescription for quetiapine," and I was like, "What?! What're you doing? I'm a *mental health nurse*, I know exactly what that is, don't give me any of that shit." Then he apologized and took it back. I don't know, he was probably getting some commission from the drug company to push it. That shit is heavy. Fuck that.'

'Does that *actually* happen?' I said, unable to hide my shock. 'Really?'

'Oh yeah, I reckon. I mean, I know I sound like a conspiracy theorist, but we had this junior doctor here for six months a few years back who was looking to be a psychiatrist. He used to legit say, "Let's quetiapine them today!" And I asked him one day why quetiapine, and he said, "They put you up in the best hotels for conferences."'

I felt sick, completely at a loss for words. Surely this didn't happen. *Surely*.

We were now standing in front of a redbrick, low-rise block of flats.

'Are we here?' I asked.

'Yup.' Aran nodded. 'This is a nice block though, not like those fake mansions back there.'

*

Merta sat in a dressing gown in her living room, cradling a cup of herbal tea in one hand and a cigarette in the other. She'd been out of hospital for two weeks, where she was held on Section 3 for almost four months. A silver tray of Jaffa Cakes sat on the polished table in front of us.

Aran was leaning forward attentively, his expression open and engaged. So different, I thought, to how he'd been with Erica and Delphi.

'I thought I wasn't psychotic at the time,' Merta was saying, 'but now, looking back, I completely *was*. I kept a notebook full of the weirdest things.' She took an elegant drag of her cigarette. Her face looked stunned, like a person perpetually caught in the flash of a camera. 'I was totally *crazy*, I'd totally snapped. I'm so frightened of ever being that way again.'

'It was very scary for you,' Aran replied, nodding.

Merta nodded back. 'I . . .' She fell silent as she put her cigarette out in a dish. Hugging her dressing gown to her body, she sat back on the sofa and looked away. 'Being sectioned was completely horrendous,' she continued, her eyes unfocused. 'It was an awful, just an *awful* place. But, I don't know, I don't want to sound ungrateful. I know I was completely . . . gone, out of my mind. I needed help. And this medication does seem to be keeping me calm. They say it's a low dose of antipsychotic – eh, risperidone it's called. And an antidepressant – I forget what now. But it seems to make me slower, so I sleep better.'

'It's helping you settle for now,' Aran said.

'Yeah, only . . .' She paused. 'Maybe I *needed* to snap, you know? To break down. To have that break from life, in a way. I was working like an addict, and things with my husband were so bad but I wasn't doing anything about it, and – does that sound stupid?'

Both Aran and I shook our heads.

'But where do I go from here?' She looked almost pleading. 'I'm so scared to actually do anything now, to change anything ever again. I'm so scared of ever having to go back *there*.'

Aran clasped his hands together. 'I know you're nervous about everything,' he said. 'I understand. You've had a bad shock. But this doesn't have to be you for ever now. This doesn't have to be your thing. You had a break, and you can get up and out of it.'

'I – *thank you*,' Merta said. 'I really appreciate hearing that.' Her eyes glassed with tears. 'Can I, um . . . can I say that the medication – it *is* helping me feel calm and sleep, but I . . . I also feel flat, kind of empty of any emotion at all. Like I'm not really here, or anywhere.' She leant forward, her voice rising. 'I'm not – *honestly* – I'm not saying I don't believe in medication. I know some people need to take it and it works really well for them. I'm grateful, I don't mean to be disrespectful. I'm just wondering why I feel sort of numb and dumb, which might not be good?' She waved her hand as if to stop us replying. 'Oh, maybe that's stupid,' she replied to herself. 'I feel so stupid, I'm sorry. I'll do whatever you say I should do.'

Aran and I looked at each other. There was a moment of knowing – knowing we both wanted to answer her, knowing how crucial this moment was for Merta, for her ability to continue to speak up and be heard. Aran smiled and raised his eyebrows. I nodded slowly, feeling deeply appreciative of him.

'You're the expert on you,' Aran said. 'Remember that. So,

we can try, carefully, to think about reducing your medication. There are risks, but there are risks either way.'

As we walked back to the office, I felt jubilant. I told Aran how much I admired his approach, and he laughed his big belly laugh. I was relieved, I told him, that there *were* people who felt a diagnosis or medication helped them, or at least initially. Though perhaps I was also relieved to relinquish my guilt momentarily, to feel purposeful. I wondered aloud if people like Merta were the lucky minority, and Aran nodded.

'The lucky ones shout the loudest,' Aran said, 'and those are the stories we hear.'

At what cost do people have their good experiences? At what cost to all those who are silenced? To those who are frightened of being called 'ungrateful', who are shouted down as 'anti-psychiatry', shamed as conspiracy theorists. Or are simply derided, and told they are *mad*?

When we got back in the office, Erica was flustered.

'What's up?' Aran asked her, putting his shoulder bag down on a desk.

Erica looked pained, her shoulders arched. 'The man I was meant to assess with Dr Evans didn't show up,' she said. 'I'm concerned, and the GP mentioned threats of violence, so I'm going to have to assess him over the phone, I think.'

'Sure, you could see if he picks up.' Aran shrugged. An immediate change in him. His cage had returned.

Erica nodded efficiently. 'Dr Evans has gone into another meeting, but I'll call him and see what I can gather.'

The man on the other end of the line talked rapidly, his

voice rising, cracking and shuddering with frustration. He explained he'd spoken to a *million different people*, that no one was taking him seriously. He spoke of the excessive noise in the flat above his own and complained that his neighbour had 'mental issues', that the man was deliberately making noise to anger him. 'I don't know *why*,' he growled. 'He's jealous of my life,' he said. 'He's trying to make everything worse for me, and I'm fucked off about it. I'm *seriously fucking angry* now. He's crazy, I tell you. He wrote on my door the other day with some weird paste, told me to fuck off.'

'Did you take a picture of the graffiti?'

'No.'

'Oh, well . . .'

The man stated that his mum had heard the noise too, but that the council didn't hear it when they came round as the neighbour had known they were there.

'But, you haven't filled in the noise diary either?' Erica asked, knowing from the GP that he hadn't.

The man mumbled something about the notebook the GP had given him to record unwelcome sounds.

'Sorry?' Erica said, her cheeks red.

'No,' he said. 'I haven't, all right? I'm too tired. He's keeping me up and I'm *so fucking tired*. I can't do shit. I can't even *SHIT* in peace.'

'So, you haven't managed to record anything or write anything down, and he was, erm, quiet when the council came round?'

'Yes! Yes!' the man yelled. 'He's making my life hell, I'm telling you that. He's got it in for me! He's got some serious mental problems! I tell you I'm going to kick his fucking head in one of these days.'

'Ah.' Erica's eyes had grown large and round in her skull. 'Now, no – please, don't do anything you'll regret later . . . when you feel . . . better. *Please*.'

'Look, someone needs to *do* something,' he pleaded. 'I'm going fucking crazy down here.'

Erica put the phone down, her eyes glazed, and left the room to find a consultant. I wondered how Erica must feel at the end of each day. Did she go over and over her assessments, the hasty decisions she was forced to make under so little guidance?

Dr Abras, who I'd only seen in passing, was in the hallway, clutching a clipboard. The four of us filed into his office.

'I'm worried,' Erica told the consultant. 'He sounds aggressive. He sounds really irate.' She relayed the conversation, peppering it with her own interpretations. 'He's quite grandiose,' she explained. 'He thinks the man's jealous of him, he's possibly elated from mania. He only really hears the noises when he's on his own there, it seems, and he's constantly calling the council and his GP. He isn't filling in the noise diary.'

'It all sounds quite paranoid,' Dr Abras said, writing something down.

Again? Surely this isn't our story again?

The doctor flicked through some notes on his computer. 'So . . . he's been stabbed in the past and was treated for PTSD, about five years ago. Quite a loner, it seems. But he isn't being treated for it any longer. Possible learning difficulties have been flagged, might be a reason for not filling in the noise diary ... but possibly he's in a state of paranoia and there *is* no noise to actually put in the diary. He certainly seems aggressive and by the sounds of it he might hurt this neighbour of his.'

Erica's brow was knitted with concern.

'So,' Dr Abras continued, 'I suggest telling his GP to prescribe an antipsychotic, possibly risperidone, but get him to tell the patient it's a medication for stress. Under the circumstances, I think it's necessary. Maybe try an SSRI antidepressant too.'

Erica nodded efficiently and turned on her heels. 'OK, will do.'

I felt my face flush, and Aran looked at me sharply from across the table, his expression stern. He shook his head. *Don't*, he mouthed. *Don't*.

The next morning I was back on the Acute Ward again. I looked for Fuad and found him in the kitchen packing away paper towels and told him the outcome for the noise man.

He leant back against the counter, folded his arms and sighed. 'Man oh *man*. The next place I'm going won't have any of that happening.'

'Oh!' I said. 'Did you get the job?'

I watched him roll the corner of a piece of paper towel between his fingers, his face empty.

'Not yet.'

'I'm sure you will,' I replied, sounding more confident than I felt.

Fuad was silent.

'Do you know Dr Evans, or Dr Abras?' I asked, pushing myself up on to the countertop across from him.

'Who?'

'Two of the consultants there.'

Fuad paused before shaking his head. 'Don't think so, but they sound like a few psychs I've known.'

'Yeah,' I said. 'I mean, I thought Delphi's assessment outcome might have been an error, but twice seems more like a general approach.'

'Oh *sure*.' Fuad rolled his eyes. 'Many of them take a risk-averse approach. There's a lot of pressure on consultants to make risky calls without having the time to really investigate.'

I considered this. *Risk-averse to whom?*

'You'd like Aran though,' I said, unsure if I had any energy to dig deeper into my thoughts.

'I've seen him around, I think. Kind of flashy?'

'Yeah.' I laughed. 'That's him.'

'OK,' Fuad said, 'let's go. There's an assessment waiting for us.'

'Oh yeah?'

We left the kitchen, passing through the hallway and into the beehive. As I turned, I noticed The Door looming. *Not long now*, I thought, *until I walk through that door for the last time.*

Fuad and I found a vacant desk and sat down. Nurses moved around us; their limbs clamouring, zigzagging trajectories, busying themselves with the business of life.

Fuad looked at me. 'You want to lead on this new admission?' He smiled widely. 'You're almost done now – with all of this. Then you can do what you need to do. So, I thought you might want to go ahead with this one, and I'll sit back – *I'll* be the student.' He smiled again and punched me lightly on the arm. 'The girl won't talk to anyone about her self-harm, so I thought maybe you could try.'

Fuad. His gentle, weathered face. His canary-yellow shirt.

'You want me to lead?' I said. I could feel my heart start to pump harder, but there was something else within me too, an unexpected steadiness.

He nodded. 'She's twenty-one, been cutting her arms and inner thighs badly. Dr Oxley's already seen her and doesn't know what to make of the self-harm. He says she's probably disassociated or psychotic, or that it's attention-seeking.' He watched me, his eyes curious. 'I thought maybe you could take another look.'

When distress has no words, no understanding or empathy for itself, it can't sit still. It is relentless, restless. An inner writhing. It is trapped, battling to get out. A horrifying, sickening unrest. It's not painful, yet it's somehow worse than pain. An indescribable turbulence – churning, squirming. Pain – physical pain – is preferable to this discomfort. And then there's that relieving *fuck it* moment. A chance to let out what's hidden, just below the surface, or deeper down – uncertain how deep. It can be a relief to cause pain. Pain is clear and focused and still. It's composed, visceral. The internal becoming external. Out. Cleansed. Gone. Through representation, the indescribable is harnessed, tamed. This momentary relief then allows for self-care, direct and clinical.

But then, just as rapid, comes the wash of guilt, of suffocating shame. The pain becomes just what it is: an ugly throb, a stain. You dislike yourself for being damaged, now more than before. You have a badge of humiliation, you fret about the practical, the mundane. You worry about infection, about your own decay. You fear you will be discarded. That you're disgusting, unloveable.

To survive life when I was younger, I sometimes harmed. I sometimes starved, and isolated. I took street drugs, going up and down and hovering above myself. I slept through everything or hardly slept. I gravitated to the people running full pelt into life, bruised and elated, or folding themselves inward, tunnelling deeper and deeper. They reflected back the parts of myself that I, in my pain, discarded. The strengths, the insights, the creative survival strategies. There was no fix, but there was *meaning*. And with meaning there was a profound change.

So, *deep breath*, I thought, standing in front of the girl's bedroom.

I pushed the door open. She was sat on a chair, her legs crossed beneath her like a pretzel. She looked up at me – *could I be different?* She smiled, her irises a brown so deep I couldn't make out the pupils at the centre.

I took a seat opposite her, and we started to talk.

9

The Exit

ON MY LUNCH BREAK I found Erica sat outside the main building. She looked pale and tired, twisting her shawl into her fists.

'Hi Erica,' I said, surprised to see her. I'd never seen her not working before. 'Are you OK?'

Erica looked past me, her eyes pink. 'That man ...' she said. Her body shuddered. 'That man with the noise ... he was assaulted this afternoon.'

I sat down on the wall beside her. She looked away.

'Who was?'

'The man with the noisy neighbour,' she said. 'The neighbour's just been arrested for physical assault on our patient.'

'Oh ... oh my God.'

'It's really bad,' she said. 'He's in a really bad way. And we were siding with the aggressor. We were calling *our* patient ill ...'

Erica rubbed at her forehead, leaving red marks in her flesh. 'And all Dr Abras said when I told him was, "So! Things will be easier for him now environment-wise." Nothing else. Nothing about the fact that we almost prescribed him an antipsychotic and diagnosed him as delusional.'

I watched Erica swivelling a ring round and round her index finger. She looked directly at me for the first time.

'I'm going to retreat back into physical medicine,' she said. 'When I finish this placement.' Her cheeks were flushed. 'It's just, to keep meeting people who've had such difficult lives, who've experienced so much – so much trauma...' She shook her head, as if ridding herself of an unpleasant image. 'Maybe it's easier for us to say "this disorder or that disorder" or, I don't know, *anything* rather than to listen to the story – the awful, overwhelming story.'

I made my way inside. The end was just weeks away now. It existed like a tear in the wallpaper which I could reach out to, peel back and climb right out of.

But there is one last person I want to tell you about.

Vera was brought on to the ward in an ambulance. She'd washed down three packets of paracetamol with vodka in her large, dilapidated home and been found by a social worker. Vera looked older than her eighty years, her body thin and flat, her discarded false teeth redundant at her side, her cheeks drawn in towards her tongue making her eyes seem disproportionally large in her ashen face. Each day she lay prostrate and resolute in the hospital bed. The curtains closed, the lights off. Any food brought to her was hurled back out the door.

'Get out, whoever you are!' she yelled at the ceiling.

I tried to talk to her.

'No!' she yelled. 'Clear off!'

On my fourth attempt, Vera let me stand just inside the door as she lay curled on top of the thin bedsheet.

'I don't feel too well,' she said to the wall.

I looked at her stringy limbs, her ghostly face. 'Can I bring you something to eat?' I asked.

Her features pinched together. 'Eat! Eat!' she spat. 'That's all anyone asks me around here!'

'I'm sorry, I . . .'

Vera sighed and turned to face the other wall. 'Just don't . . .' She trailed off. 'Please don't let me live to be ancient. How can people *do* this? Am I a criminal? I did nothing to anybody but myself. When will this torment be over?'

Slowly, over the next few days, Vera began to talk. I would settle on the chair beside her bed while she lay there, knees tucked into her hollow frame, socks slipping off her thin feet, strands of hair plastered to her forehead with sweat.

'This is the same hospital that ruined her,' Vera whispered. 'This is where she was turned into a zombie.' She snapped her head round to glare at me. '*No*,' she growled, 'I won't take *any* of their filth, not one single tablet! I've seen what it did to Beth.'

'Who was Beth, Vera?'

'Beth, my sister.'

'Your sister was here?'

'Yes, this hospital. We took her here – well, we allowed her to be here. Many, many years ago now. More than fifty, I think. I – let her come here.'

'You must have been worried about her?' I tried.

Vera was silent for a while. 'We were, all of us were – back then,' she said carefully. 'Beth was always different, you know. Opinionated, angry. Her rages at our father – he really hated her sometimes. I could never really . . . I don't know what really happened, but she could scare me. Then everyone said she was ill.'

Vera's face was wet with tears. She wiped them away on her pillow.

'It must have been hard to know what to do,' I offered.

She licked at a tear near the corner of her mouth. 'She seemed so . . . unhappy. After she came out of here, something had just *changed*. Something snuffed right out in her. She wasn't angry any more, but she also wasn't *anything* any more. Then after that she wouldn't leave her bed. We had to carry her out and wash her, sit her on the toilet – you can imagine. She just stared at my parents – hateful stares. And me too. I was holding out her pills in my palm, pushing them into her mouth, begging her to swallow them. I didn't *know*. I think she tried so many times to tell me things, but I was young, I didn't understand. I thought I was making her better, even though something didn't feel right to me.'

I watched Vera curled up on the bed. And now she too was here, replicating her sister's stagnant protest.

'I feel terrible,' she continued. 'So, so guilty to be still alive when she's not. I don't deserve it. I don't deserve to be happy when she wasn't. I don't deserve a different fate from hers.' Vera's knees rose higher towards her chin. Her eyes closed.

There was a knock on the door, and Vera's head snapped round at a speed so at odds with her lethargy that I jumped.

'Vera, hello!' someone called from the other side. 'I was hoping to catch you today.' The door began to open, and I saw a flash of orange coat, a face.

'I said GET OUT!' Vera yelled. 'Get OUT of my room!'

The woman quickly shut the door. I could hear her apologizing, telling Vera she'd be back again soon.

'This blasted social worker,' Vera said, rearranging her head on the pillow. 'It's taken her too long! Where was she at Christmas when I had no food and no company? My house falling down around me. Dropping in once a month, was she? No thanks. I don't trust her. She can bugger off.'

The days ticked by, and each day Vera became stiller, smaller. Staff began avoiding her room. She stopped eating and drinking, her skin taking on a pallid, moist look. Her eyes like two broken headlamps.

'Hopefully I'll be dead soon,' she said. 'I'll be nothing but skin and bone.' She turned, suddenly forceful. 'Oh, why won't you just leave me alone to die? That's all I deserve.'

The next afternoon when I went into Vera's room, I distractedly left her door open behind me.

There in the doorway stood Rich. His gloved hands, his camo jacket, his sunglasses. He pointed two invisible pistols into the room.

Vera sat up like she'd been burnt with a poker. I shot her a panicked look, thinking she was going to launch a cup of water across at him.

Rich slid his sunglasses calmly on to his head, revealing his dark-ringed eyes. 'Ma'am, ma'am,' he said, nodding at each of us in turn.

Vera was silent. She tilted her head and peered at him. Rich remained in the doorway, his eyes fixed on the tiny, frail woman on the bed before him.

'Rich,' I said slowly, 'this is Vera.'

Rich took my words as a prompt to start inspecting the doorframe like a carpenter. Vera, still silent, watched him.

'Need any work done here to keep them out?' he said to the wood. 'Could do with a bit of a touch-up. Some better protection all round for you.'

I studied Vera closely, feeling my chest expanding and falling.

'Hmm,' Vera said, her eyes squinting. The fine hairs on her upper lip were damp.

'Can't be too careful,' Rich said, taking off a glove and feeling over the wood again with his bare hand. 'And I'm the only one on duty round here.'

'Can you . . . keep everyone out of here?' Vera asked him, still squinting.

'Sure,' Rich replied, nonchalantly. 'I can guard you if you like.'

Without warning, he strode into the room and reached out his gloveless hand to Vera. To my surprise, she raised a stringy arm and shook it. 'Hello there, young man,' she said softly, looking deep into his face.

I watched as they inspected each other, their hands intertwined.

Rich let his fingers slip gently from hers before moving

towards the window. He dropped down to peer closely at the ledge. 'I could look into sealing all this up too, if you like,' he said. 'They can get in the tiniest cracks.'

Vera was smiling. 'Thank you,' she murmured. 'You're a lovely boy.' Her eyes followed him.

Rich said nothing, but I noticed his cheeks were pink.

'What're you doing in this place?' Vera asked, pulling herself into a seated position.

'Oh,' replied Rich, looking away, 'I'm not well, you see. I've got to get *fully well* before I can go home.'

We sat in silence as Rich wiped at the glass with his glove and peered out into the empty courtyard beyond.

'I'll be back later,' he said, turning from us. 'I'll make sure you're secure.'

Vera thanked him and watched him go.

'A nice man,' she murmured. 'Poor man ... someone should be taking care of him.' She looked over at me. 'Does he have any family? Do they visit?'

'No,' I said, 'his family don't seem to visit.' I immediately wondered if I shouldn't have shared this.

'That's sad,' she said quietly, shaking her head. 'Well ... well. Why's he telling himself that about being ill? He seems all right to me. Who's flipping *well* these days?'

The room was still. I watched Vera staring at her knees, and thought how grateful I was for Rich's unaffected disruption.

'You were kind to him,' I said. 'You have a very caring way.'

I meant it. Something had been freed from her in that moment, something luminescent.

Vera closed her eyes momentarily, before turning towards me. 'I do like to help, I suppose. I don't like to see anyone on their own, anyone sad.' She looked past me. 'Do you think you could open that window a little?'

Later that evening, Vera accepted a sandwich and black coffee.

The next day she called a senior nurse into her room and asked to appeal her section. The nurse, astonished, agreed to start the process for a tribunal.

*

A tribunal has the power to release you from your section. If you are detained under Section 2, Section 3 or Section 37, you can take your chances at the court. There are time restrictions which you have to meet when applying, and you must consider your timings carefully. On Section 2, you have the right to appeal within fourteen days. If you are detained under Section 3, you can appeal to a tribunal only once in the first six months. If it fails, you can apply just once within each six-month renewal period.

A tribunal is usually a panel of three people: a solicitor or a barrister, a psychiatrist who is not your usual clinician, and a lay member of the public with mental health experience. They sit alongside the patient, a nurse, the patient's psychiatrist, a social worker and an optional family member. Reports are exchanged, evidence given, questions asked and reassessments arranged. You can represent yourself and state your case, or you can request help. The tribunal then decides if you should be discharged from your section under the Mental Health Act, or carry on serving it.

*

In the days leading up to the tribunal, Vera ate heartily. She talked with Rich and left her room with the help of her new walking aid, a momentum and purpose to her movements. She shook her fist at grievances, and rallied other patients outside the doctor's office.

'To hell with that!' she exclaimed.

'What hot shit is this?' she protested.

On the morning of the tribunal, Vera was awake and sat on the edge of her bed when I started my shift at seven. She had repositioned her teeth, and her full cheeks were glowing.

I'd borrowed a wheelchair, knowing the tribunal was being held in another part of the hospital, and hoped she'd agree to let me take her there.

'Goodness,' she said, looking at the chair as I wheeled it in, 'am I *that* old?'

We both laughed.

'I wasn't sure you'd fully got your strength back yet,' I said.

'Hmm, *well*.' She smiled. 'I'll pretend I'm royalty being chaperoned.'

As I pushed her along the hallway past the day area, Vera spun around towards me and clasped my arm. Her face was stretched and panicked. 'You're *coming with me*, right?'

I looked around for someone to ask, but there was just me. A nearly-nurse. I nodded. 'Sure.'

During the trial Vera was articulate and challenging, sitting rod-straight in her chair. She made an eloquent case for her release, highlighting poor care and inconsistencies in decisions. The visiting clinician seemed to take an instant dislike to Dr Oxley, who appeared sullen and monosyllabic throughout. His brow sank lower and lower as Vera spoke. The decision was unanimous, and Vera won the right to leave the ward. The panel instructed that suitable residential housing be found so that she be less isolated at home.

As we wheeled out of the room, Vera's headlight-eyes were flickering brighter than I'd ever seen them.

'I'm not *any* of the nonsense that Oxley says I am,' she said. 'I'm just a human being figuring it out as I go along.'

When we got back to the ward, she sat at a table in the day area and drank coffee, making chit-chat with passing staff and patients. Beside her, I sipped my tea as the room filled up for dinner. A line had begun to form. I watched, not wanting to forget a single second of anything, anyone. *What stories have we told ourselves?* I thought. *And do these stories bind us in time, or carry us forward with hope?*

Vera was watching me. There was a tear on her cheek. 'If this is help,' she said, slowly, 'then God help the world. I feel sorry for all these young-uns – the poor buggers. At least it doesn't matter all that much for me.' She put her cup down.

In another room, someone was shouting. An alarm began to shriek.

'You need to learn from this,' she said. 'Learn, and do it bloody better.'

Epilogue

When I began reading voraciously as a teenager, I empathized deeply with characters labelled 'mad', silenced by those around them to obfuscate the mirror they held up to an unwelcome reality. Looking back, I recognize that they spoke to my own story: the wordlessness surrounding my parents' emotional volatility and struggles with addiction within the performative exterior that existed for friends and family. These 'mad' characters articulated both my shame and desire to be seen, to be less alone. They illuminated a duplicitous adult world where the exposure of contentious truths threatened the delicate balance of our constructed lives.

Decades later, I'm questioning what role psychiatry plays in silencing those who hold a mirror up to what we wish desperately to ignore.

I have written this book in the hope that readers will be shocked out of their trust and complacency for our current system, and move towards action.

Publicly criticizing psychiatry and our treatment of mental ill health is terrifying. It is an issue that fuels vehement responses which can cloud our ability to hear each other and drive us to lash out and attack. Exploration of this topic reaches deep into our unconscious. It threatens our understanding of ourselves, and our relationship with the world. It magnifies our ability to repress and ignore the things that are too painful to confront.

I'm aware that I don't know how you, the reader, will react to what you've just read. I know that these stories can stir up rage, disbelief and denial. They did in me. I know how it feels to be sat opposite a tutor or clinician and be shaking with emotion as you try to get the words out. I know how it feels to be overwhelmed and demoralized, or driven unequivocally to act.

I can't know how this book has affected you, but I can hope that it helps people with similar experiences to speak up and be believed, both the survivors of psychiatric treatment and the staff who resist the pressure to conform.

The continuing rise in hospital admissions, in suicides and violence and deaths, in prescriptions for psychiatric drugs, tells us our system is *not* working. In 2023 the NHS spent approximately £629 million on psychiatric drugs, and funding and focus within mental health research continues to be on medication. Meanwhile, there are cuts for social and psychological support – emotional, familial, practical, financial – the areas that impact our mental wellbeing the most. The waiting lists for talking therapies across the NHS and within the charity sector continue to grow, with offerings that are increasingly short-term, generic and mechanistic.

Alternative services do exist, though they remain rare. They are not given adequate funding, and continue to be marginalized. Peers within the NHS are largely poorly paid and undervalued, and those who question treatment plans or professional opinions are often weeded out as 'troublemakers'. There are, however, unique NHS teams working in radical ways within the constraints of the system. Alex, just a few years on from his training, now co-runs one of these teams. His anger and hope still burn brightly. Fuad finally got a job in The Garden, a therapeutic ward focusing on holistic treatment and medication reduction. And Nia left her post as a peer in the community team to work as a low-cost psychotherapist.

I think daily about the patients I met across my two years training within the NHS, and wish I knew where life has taken them. I hope they are safe, and no longer within the tunnels of psychiatry.

I still feel some shame that I was too crushed to stay within the system. Though I now feel honoured to work alongside individuals both with and without a diagnosis, helping them to validate and make sense of their own narrative and their relationship to medication or to a diagnosis, and to centre their own experiences, opinions and needs.

Because, in mental health, the 'expert' is not the clinician in the white coat or the cardigan, it is *you*. Madness and emotional distress can and should be temporary; it is a meaningful crisis filled with the potential for change, for hope.

It's not easy to live 'well' or to find meaning. When we are overwhelmed by distressing thoughts and experiences our current system tells us we are defective – mentally, chemically. That by handing ourselves over to a professional, by being passive, 'good' patients, we will be fixed. Psychiatry does *to* us, rather than works *with* us.

Yet, mental distress or ill health is not the same as a broken leg. We cannot get fully well – whatever that means to us – without considering that our distress contains *meaning*. Distress tells us something about our lives. A 'symptom' is threaded through with personal stories and traumas, our losses and fears, the societal barriers and discriminations that have plagued us. If we are aided early on to explore and acknowledge these threads, to heal from them, distress can be a map which enables us to live differently.

There is a narrative we've become comfortable with, which most of us digest without feeling or action: *Mental health services are underfunded and understaffed.*

But this is only half the story. The other half is messy and confronting. It is philosophical and systemic. It is uncomfortable enough to make us look sharply away. But it is this part that we urgently need to acknowledge if things are to truly change.

Our mental health services are *also* underfunded and understaffed. But to endorse this as the only problem is not just a plaster on a gaping wound, but obfuscating the truth.

There are a growing number of individuals – psychiatric survivors, staff, academics – fighting enormous battles within and around psychiatry. Unimaginable leaps of progress are happening in the wings. Progress that every one of us can be part of, through the questions we ask, the curiosity we show, how we protect ourselves and our loved ones. Through our demand for more, for better.

We can learn from this. Learn, and do it bloody better.

Terminology in the UK System

Mental health nurse / psychiatric nurse
Interchangeable terms for a nurse with a specialism in mental health, whether working in a community team or ward setting.

Psychiatric liaison nurse
A mental health nurse who works in a general hospital across wards and A&E to provide psychiatric assessment and brief treatment.

Psychiatrist
A medical doctor who has specialized in assessing, diagnosing and treating mental illness/mental health, largely by focusing on targeting the symptoms of the condition they have diagnosed by prescribing medication. They can also make referrals to psychologists, therapy groups, psychotherapists or social workers. They generally have very limited training in talking therapy, and studies show that the number of psychiatrists using talking therapy with patients has declined rapidly over the last twenty years.

Medical psychotherapists
A psychiatrist who has also undergone full psychotherapy training. This speciality is very rare. In 2021, there were just thirty-two consultants in medical psychotherapy working in the NHS in England.

Peer support worker
A staff member or volunteer who uses their personal experience of living with a condition to help others on their recovery journey through advice, befriending, assistance, training and workshops.

Health care assistant / health care support worker
A staff member who supports clinical care, monitoring and chaperoning.

Psychologists / counselling psychologists / clinical psychologists / forensic psychologists, etc.
Psychologists study human emotion, thoughts and behaviour and work with people to change and improve the way they think, act and interact. They are either 'research-oriented' – furthering knowledge of the mind through scientific study – or 'applied' – working therapeutically with people by largely focusing on changing thoughts and behaviour to reduce distress and improve emotional and practical functioning. They may work in a solution-focused, goal-oriented way or use interventions to navigate past experiences and traumas. Psychologists are also trained to assess and diagnose mental health conditions, and often work closely with psychiatrists.

Psychotherapists / psychotherapeutic counsellors / counsellors / psychoanalysts, etc.

Psychotherapists largely work longer-term with people, and are trained in various psychological theories and intervention techniques. They usually support a person to delve into the complex web of causes for mental distress and/or illness, focusing both on the here and now, as well as stretching back into past experiences and their unconscious impact. Psychotherapists aim to help a person to make long-lasting changes to their relationship with themselves and others. In general, they do not work through the lens of psychiatric diagnostic categories, instead focusing on the person's understanding of themselves.

The composite environments

The ward is a composite of three wards across nine months.

In general, psychiatric wards are split into male and female wards, as well as wards for children up to eighteen years old, adults from eighteen to sixty-five, and older adults from sixty-six.

The Community Treatment Team is a composite of three teams across six months.

A&E is a composite of two teams across five months.

Further Reading, Support and Advice

BOOKS

Davies, James, *Cracked: Why Psychiatry is Doing More Harm Than Good* (Icon Books, 2013)

Fernando, Suman, *Mental Health, Race and Culture* (3rd ed.) (Red Globe Press, 2010)

Filer, Nathan, *This Book Will Change Your Mind About Mental Health: A Journey into the Heartland of Psychiatry* (Faber & Faber, 2019)

Frazer-Carroll, Micha, *Mad World: The Politics of Mental Health* (Pluto Press, 2023)

Geekie, Jim, Randal, Patte, Lampshire, Debra and Read, John (eds), *Experiencing Psychosis: Personal and Professional Perspectives* (Routledge, 2011)

Harewood, David, *Maybe I Don't Belong Here: A Memoir of Race, Identity, Breakdown and Recovery* (Bluebird, 2022)

Hari, Johann, *Lost Connections: Why You're Depressed and How to Find Hope* (Bloomsbury, 2018)

Johnstone, Lucy, *A Straight Talking Introduction to Psychiatric Diagnosis* (2nd ed.) (PCCS Books, 2022)

Linton, Samara and Walcott, Rianna, *The Colour of Madness: 65 Voices Reflect on Race and Mental Health* (Bluebird, 2024)

Moncrieff, Joanna, *A Straight Talking Introduction to Psychiatric Drugs: The Truth About How They Work and How to Come Off Them* (2nd ed.) (PCCS Books, 2020)

Rapley, Mark, Moncrieff, Joanna and Dillon, Jacqui (eds), *De-medicalizing Misery: Psychiatry, Psychology and the Human Condition* (Palgrave Macmillan, 2011)

Russo, Jasna and Sweeney, Angela (eds), *Searching for a Rose Garden: Challenging Psychiatry, Fostering Mad Studies* (PCCS Books, 2016)

Watson, Jo (ed.), *Drop the Disorder!: Challenging the Culture of Psychiatric Diagnosis* (PCCS Books, 2019)

WEBSITES AND BLOGS

Asylum Magazine (https://asylummagazine.org/) – a forum for free and open debate about controversial issues in mental health and psychiatry

Black Mental Health Workers Alliance (https://www.bmhwa.co.uk/) – coalition of carers, practitioners and people with lived experience fighting for systemic change

Dolly Sen (www.dollysen.com) – activist for change in psychiatry

Fireweed Collective (https://fireweedcollective.org) – grassroots network that looks beyond the medical model

Hearing Voices Network (www.hearing-voices.org) – information and advice for people who hear voices or have visions

I Got Better (www.igotbetter.org) – stories of recovery

Laura Delano (www.lauradelano.com) – a story of recovery

Mad in America / Mad in the UK (www.madinamerica.com / www.madintheuk.com) – critical perspectives on all aspects of mental health

National Survivor User Network (www.nsun.org.uk) – a service user-led charity aiming to shape policy and services, with groups and resources

Open Dialogue (https://opendialogueapproach.co.uk/) – a social network model of mental healthcare and treatment

Rachel Waddingham (www.behindthelabel.co.uk) – a story of recovery

The Council for Evidence-Based Psychiatry (www.cepuk.org) – critical evaluation of psychiatric practice

The Critical Mental Health Nurses Network (https://criticalmh-nursing.org) – promoting critical thinking about the practice and culture of mental health nursing

The Inner Compass (www.theinnercompass.org) – resources about psychiatric drugs

The International Institute for Psychiatric Drug Withdrawal (https://iipdw.org/) – support, research and training about psychiatric drug withdrawal

The Power Threat Meaning Framework (www.bps.org.uk/power-threat-meaning-framework) – alternative to the medical model of distress

The Soteria Network (https://www.soterianetwork.org.uk/) – supporting the development of non-medical alternatives to psychiatric services across the UK

The Voices in My Head (www.ted.com/talks/eleanor_longden_the_voices_in_my_head) – short TED talk: Eleanor Longden talks about her experiences in psychiatric services

Voice Collective (www.voicecollective.co.uk) – for young people who hear, see and sense things that others don't

RESEARCH

Autism and misdiagnosis

1. Darling Rasmussen, P. (2022), '"I was never broken – I just don't fit in this world": A case report series of misdiagnosed women with higher functioning ASD', *Nordic Journal of Psychiatry*, 77(4), 352–359.
2. Allely, C. S., Woodhouse, E., Mukherjee, R. A. (2023), 'Autism spectrum disorder and personality disorders: How do clinicians carry out a differential diagnosis?', *Autism*, 27(6), 1847–1850.
3. Kentrou, V., Livingston, L. A., Grove, R. et al (2024), 'Perceived misdiagnosis of psychiatric conditions in autistic adults', *eClinicalMedicine*, Apr, 71(4).

4. Au-Yeung, S. K., Bradley, L., Robertson, A. E. et al (2019), 'Experience of mental health diagnosis and perceived misdiagnosis in autistic, possibly autistic and non-autistic adults', *Autism*, 23(6), 1508–1518.
5. Van Schalkwyk, G. I., Peluso, F., Qayyum, Z. et al (2015), 'Varieties of Misdiagnosis in ASD: An Illustrative Case Series', *Journal of Autism and Developmental Disorders*, 45, 911–918.
6. Iversen, S., Kildahl, A. N. (2022), 'Case Report: Mechanisms in Misdiagnosis of Autism as Borderline Personality Disorder', *Frontiers in Psychology*, 13:735205.
7. Ying, Jiangbo, Zhang, M. W., Sajith, S. G. (2023), 'Misdiagnosis of Psychosis and Obsessive-Compulsive Disorder in a Young Patient with Autism Spectrum Disorder', *Case Reports in Psychiatry*, 5.

ECT

1. Read, J. (2022), 'A response to yet another defence of ECT in the absence of robust efficacy and safety evidence', *Epidemiology and Psychiatric Sciences*, Feb, 15;31:e13.
2. Oppenheim, M. (2022), 'Thousands of women given "dangerous" electric shocks as mental health treatment in England', *Independent*, 19 June.
3. Read, J., Bentall, R. (2010), 'The effectiveness of electroconvulsive therapy: A literature review', *Epidemiologia e Psichiatria Sociale*, Dec, 19(4):333–347.
4. Fosse, R., Read, J. (2013), 'Electroconvulsive Treatment: Hypotheses about Mechanisms of Action', *Frontiers in Psychiatry*, 4, 94.
5. Rose, D., Fleischmann, P., Wykes, T. et al (2003), 'Patients' perspectives on electroconvulsive therapy: systematic review', *British Medical Journal*, 326:1363.
6. Read, J., Moncrieff, J. (2022), 'Depression: why drugs and electricity are not the answer', *Psychological Medicine*, 52(8).

FURTHER READING, SUPPORT AND ADVICE

Psychiatric drugs used in dementia

1. Alzheimer's Society website (2025): https://www.alzheimers.org.uk/about-dementia/treatments/drugs/antipsychotic-drugs
2. Macfarlane, S., Cunningham, C. (2021), 'Limiting antipsychotic drugs in dementia', *Australian Prescriber*, Feb, 44(1): 8–11.
3. King's College London, News Centre (2014): https://www.kcl.ac.uk/news/spotlight/reducing-the-use-of-antipsychotics-in-dementia
4. Cosgrave, A. (2024), 'Antipsychotics for dementia linked to more harms than previously acknowledged', Alzheimer's Research Centre, 18 Apr.
5. Mok, P. L. H., Carr, M. J., Guthrie B. et al (2024), 'Multiple adverse outcomes associated with antipsychotic use in people with dementia: population based matched cohort study', *British Medical Journal*, 385.
6. Rogowska, M., Thornton, M., Creese, B. et al (2023), 'Implications of Adverse Outcomes Associated with Antipsychotics in Older Patients with Dementia: A 2011–2022 Update', *Drugs Aging*, Jan, 40(1): 21–32.
7. Rochon, P. A., Vozoris, N., Gill, S. (2017), 'The harms of benzodiazepines for patients with dementia', *Canadian Medical Association Journal*, 10 Apr, 189 (14).
8. Stevenson, D. G. et al (2010), 'Antipsychotic and Benzodiazepine Use Among Nursing Home Residents: Findings from the 2004 National Nursing Home Survey', *American Journal of Geriatric Psychiatry*, Volume 18, Issue 12, 1078–1092.

Racism and bias

1. Mind website, facts and figures about racism and mental health: www.mind.org.uk/about-us/our-strategy/becoming-a-truly-anti-racist-organisation/

2. King, C. et al (2021), 'From Preproduction to Coproduction: COVID-19, whiteness, and making black mental health matter', *The Lancet Psychiatry*, Volume 8, Issue 2, 93–95.
3. King, C., Jeynes, T. (2021), 'Mad Studies Birmingham: Whiteness, madness, and reform of the Mental Health Act', *The Lancet Psychiatry*, Jun, 8(6): 460–461.
4. Beresford, P., Rose, D. (2023), 'Decolonising global mental health: The role of Mad Studies', *Global Mental Health*, 26 May, 10.
5. Widge A. S., Jordan, A., Kraguljac, N. V. et al (2023), 'Structural Racism in Psychiatric Research Careers: Eradicating Barriers to a More Diverse Workforce', *American Journal of Psychiatry*, 1 Sept, 180 (9): 645–659.
6. Antić, A. (2021), 'Transcultural Psychiatry: Cultural Difference, Universalism and Social Psychiatry in the Age of Decolonisation', *Culture, Medicine and Psychiatry*, Sept, 45(3): 359–384.
7. Dixon, J., Wilkinson-Tough, M., Stone, K., Laing, J. (2019), 'Treading a tightrope: Professional perspectives on balancing the rights of patients and relatives under the Mental Health Act in England', *Health and Social Care in the Community*, 28(1), 300–308.
8. Future Care Capital – organization focused on transformation of health and care provision (Feb 2024), 'Black mental health inpatients more likely to be forcibly restrained by police' (https://futurecarecapital.org.uk/latest/black-inpatients-more-forcibly-restrained/).
9. NHS England, Mental Health Act Statistics, Annual Figures 2020–21 (https://digital.nhs.uk/data-and-information/publications/statistical/mental-health-act-statistics-annual-figures/).
10. NHS Archives – statistics in mental health (https://webarchive.nationalarchives.gov.uk/).
11. Townsend, E. (24 November 2022), '"Staggering" rise in restraint of black people in mental healthcare', *Health Service Journal* (news, analysis and data about the UK healthcare system), https://www.hsj.co.uk/
12. Faber, S. C., Khanna Roy, A., Michaels, T. I., Williams, M. T. (2023), 'The weaponization of medicine: Early psychosis in the Black

community and the need for racially informed mental healthcare', *Frontiers in Psychiatry*, 9 Feb, 14.
13. The Synergi Collaborative Centre: Initiative to reframe, rethink and transform realities of ethnic inequalities in mental illness (https://legacy.synergicollaborativecentre.co.uk/briefing-papers/)
14. Nazroo, J. Y., Rhodes, J. (2020), 'Where next for understanding race/ethnic inequalities in severe mental illness? Structural, interpersonal and institutional racism', *Sociology of Health & Illness*, Vol. 42, No. 2.

CLINICAL SUPERVISION AND SAFE CARE

1. McCarron, R. H., Eade, J., Delmage, E. (2018), 'The experience of clinical supervision for nurses and healthcare assistants in a secure adolescent service: Affecting service improvement', *Journal of Psychiatric and Mental Health Nursing*, Apr, 25(3).
2. Marshman, C., Hansen, A., Munro, I. (2022), 'Compassion fatigue in mental health nurses: A systematic review', *Journal of Psychiatric and Mental Health Nursing*, 29, 529–543.
3. Bradley, W. J., Becker, K. D. (2021), 'Clinical supervision of mental health services: a systematic review of supervision characteristics and practices associated with formative and restorative outcomes', *Clinical Supervisor*, 40(1), 88–111.
4. Rothwell, C., Kehoe, A., Farook, S. F. et al (2021), 'Enablers and barriers to effective clinical supervision in the workplace: a rapid evidence review', *BMJ Open*, 11.
5. Allan, R., McLuckie, A., Hoffecker, L. (2017), 'PROTOCOL: Effects of clinical supervision of mental health professionals on supervisee knowledge, skills, attitudes and behaviour, and client outcomes: protocol for a systematic review', *Campbell Systematic Reviews*, 13: 1–44.
6. Edwards, D., Burnard, P., Hannigan, B. et al (2006), 'Clinical supervision and burnout: the influence of clinical supervision for

community mental health nurses', *Journal of Clinical Nursing*, 15: 1007–1015.
7. White, E., Winstanley, J. (2021), 'Clinical supervision provided to mental health nurses in England', *British Journal of Mental Health Nursing*, 10:2, 1–11.

CLOZAPINE

1. De Leon, J. (2022), 'According to the WHO clozapine pharmacovigilance database, the United Kingdom accounts for 968 fatal outcomes versus 892 in the rest of the world', *British Journal of Clinical Pharmacology*, 88: 5434–5435.
2. De las Cuevas, C., Sanz, E. J., De Leon, J. (2024), 'Adverse drug reactions and their fatal outcomes in clozapine patients in VigiBase: Comparing the top four reporting countries (US, UK, Canada and Australia)', *Schizophrenia Research*, 268, 165–174.
3. De Leon, J., Ruan C. J., Schoretsanitis, G., De las Cuevas, C. (2020), 'A Rational Use of Clozapine Based on Adverse Drug Reactions, Pharmacokinetics, and Clinical Pharmacopsychology', *Psychotherapy and Psychosomatics*, 89(4): 200–214.
4. Henderson, D. C. et al (2005), 'Clozapine, Diabetes Mellitus, Hyperlipidemia, and Cardiovascular Risks and Mortality: Results of a 10-Year Naturalistic Study', *Journal of Clinical Psychiatry*, 66(9): 1116–1121.
5. Centre for Evidence-Based Medicine (2024): 'What role has epidemiologist Georgia Richard's Preventable Deaths Tracker played in establishing if Clozapine is Britain's most dangerous prescription drug?'
6. Dyer, C. (2018), 'Coroners warn health secretary of clozapine deaths', *British Medical Journal*, 363.
7. *Guardian* (2018), 'Coroners urge health secretary to ensure that clozapine, linked to two deaths, does not claim more lives'.
8. Buckley, N. A., Sanders, P. (2000), 'Cardiovascular Adverse Effects of Antipsychotic Drugs', *Drug-Safety*, 23, 215–228.
9. De Hert, M., Detraux, J. et al (2012), 'Metabolic and cardiovascular

adverse effects associated with antipsychotic drugs', *Nature Reviews Endocrinology*, 8, 114–126.
10. Haas, S. J., Hill, R. et al (2007), 'Clozapine-Associated Myocarditis', *Drug-Safety*, 30, 47–57.
11. De las Cuevas, C. et al (2024), 'Revealing the reporting disparity: VigiBase highlights underreporting of clozapine in other Western European countries compared to the UK', *Schizophrenia Research*, 268, 175–188.

TARDIVE DYSKINESIA

1. Kim, J., Macmaster, E., Schwartz, T. L. (2014), 'Tardive dyskinesia in patients treated with atypical antipsychotics: Case series and brief review of etiologic and treatment considerations', *Drugs Context*, 9 Apr, 3.
2. Carbon, M., Kane J. M., Leucht, S. et al (2018), 'Tardive dyskinesia risk with first- and second-generation antipsychotics in comparative randomized controlled trials: a meta-analysis', *World Psychiatry*, Oct, 17(3), 330–340.
3. Leucht, S., Wahlbeck, K. et al (2003), 'New generation antipsychotics versus low-potency conventional antipsychotics: a systematic review and meta-analysis', *Lancet*, 10 May, 361.
4. Solmi, M., Pigato, G., Kane, J. M., Correll, C. (2018), 'Clinical risk factors for the development of tardive dyskinesia', *Journal of the Neurological Sciences*, 389, 21–27.
5. 'Tardive Dyskinesia Facts and Figures', *Psychiatric Times*, 30 May 2019 (https://www.psychiatrictimes.com/view/tardive-dyskinesia-facts-and-figures).
6. Wonodi, I., Reeves, G., Carmichael, D. et al (2007), 'Tardive dyskinesia in children treated with atypical antipsychotic medications', *Movement Disorders*, 15 Sept, 22(12)
7. Caroff, S. N. (2019), 'Overcoming barriers to effective management of tardive dyskinesia', *Neuropsychiatric Disease and Treatment*, 4 Apr, 15: 785–794.

8. 'Neurocrine Biosciences Raises Awareness of Tardive Dyskinesia and its Impact on Patients', 6 May 2019 (https://www.biospace.com/neurocrine-biosciences-honors-mental-health-month-and-raises-awareness-of-tardive-dyskinesia-and-its-impact-on-patients).

PSYCHIATRIC POLYPHARMACY AND OVERPRESCRIBING

1. Allott, K., Pert, A., Rattray, A., Cooper, R. E., Winther Davy, J., Grünwald, L., Horowitz, M., Moncrieff, J. et al (2024), 'An ethics analysis of antipsychotic dose reduction and discontinuation: Principles for supporting recovery from psychosis', *Psychiatric Rehabilitation Journal*, 47(4), 291–302.
2. Guy, A., Brown, M., Lewis, S., Horowitz, M. (2020), 'The "patient voice": patients who experience antidepressant withdrawal symptoms are often dismissed, or misdiagnosed with relapse, or a new medical condition', *Therapeutic Advances in Psychopharmacology*, 9 Nov, 10.
3. Jerjes, W., Ramsay, D., Stevenson, H., Lalji, K. (2024), 'Mental Health Polypharmacy in "Non-Coded" Primary Care Patients: The Effect of Deprescribing', *Journal of Clinical Medicine*, 7 Feb, 13(4): 958.
4. Silvernail, C. M., Wright, S. L. (2022), 'Surviving Benzodiazepines: A Patient's and Clinician's Perspectives', *Advanced Therapeutics*, May, 39(5): 1871–1880.
5. Soerensen, A., Nielsen, L., Poulsen, B. K. et al (2016), 'Potentially inappropriate prescriptions in patients admitted to a psychiatric hospital', *Nordic Journal of Psychiatry*, Jul, 70(5): 365–373.
6. 'Deprescribing in mental health: pragmatic steps for a better quality of life', *Journal of Prescribing Practice* (2021) (https://www.prescribingpractice.com/content/better-practice/deprescribing-in-mental-health-pragmatic-steps-for-a-better-quality-of-life/).
7. Read, J., Gee, A., Diggle, J., Butler, H. (2017), 'The interpersonal adverse effects reported by 1008 users of antidepressants; and the incremental impact of polypharmacy', *Psychiatry Research*, 256, 423–427.

8. Davies, J., Cooper, R. E., Moncrieff, J., Montagu, L. et al (2022), 'The costs incurred by the NHS in England due to the unnecessary prescribing of dependency-forming medications', *Addictive Behaviors*, Volume 125.
9. Turabian, J. (2021), 'Psychotropic Drugs Originate Permanent Biological Changes that Go Against Resolution of Mental Health Problems: A View from the General Medicine', *Journal of Addictive Disorders and Mental Health*.
10. Ito, H., Koyama, A., Higuchi, T. (2005), 'Polypharmacy and excessive dosing: Psychiatrists' perceptions of antipsychotic drug prescription', *British Journal of Psychiatry*, 187(3): 243–247.
11. Valtonen, J., Karrasch, M. (2020), 'Polypharmacy-induced cognitive dysfunction and discontinuation of psychotropic medication: a neuropsychological case report', *Therapeutic Advances in Psychopharmacology*, 10.
12. Horowitz, M. A., Kelleher, M., Taylor, D. (2021), 'Should gabapentinoids be prescribed long-term for anxiety and other mental health conditions?', *Addictive Behaviors*, Volume 119.
13. Zhang, C., Spence, O., Reeves, G. et al (2020), 'Characteristics of youths treated with psychotropic polypharmacy in the United States, 1999 to 2015', *JAMA Pediatrics*, 2 Nov.
14. Read, J. (2022), 'How important are informed consent, informed choice, and patient-doctor relationships, when prescribing antipsychotic medication?', *Journal of Mental Health*, 34(1), 4–12.

REDACTING RECORDS OF MENTAL HEALTH PATIENTS

1. https://www.england.nhs.uk/long-read/redacting-information-for-online-record-access/

NHS SPENDING FIGURES ON PSYCHIATRIC DRUGS

1. 5 Dec 2024: 'latest mental health medicine statistics' (https://media.nhsbsa.nhs.uk/press-releases/).

Acknowledgements

My incredible agent, Anna Dixon, for picking this manuscript out of the bin, for your deep empathy for the people depicted and your fantastic ideas. It wouldn't exist without you.

My visionary editor, Sharika Teelwah, for your trust and bravery in taking a shot on something so complex, your truly insightful and kind edits, and your ability to understand what I was trying to say before even I knew.

My friends, the generous and talented readers, editors and encouragers: David Anderson, Jay Chakravorty, Emma Hooper, Jonathan Gadsby, and most especially Lucy Fernandes – you're an inspiration. This book couldn't have been written without your support and constantly enlightening, humanizing input.

Dan Balado, for your thoughtful and sensitive copy edits.

Lucy Johnstone, for the wise teachings and reassurance which saw me through my training.

Daniel Langley, for the unending fight, for the hope.

Camilla Gugenheim, for listening.

Jono, for all the thousands of conversations and tears, for your confidence in me and this project, for reading and editing countless terrible drafts, for holding me together through it all, and for absolutely everything else I can't put into words.

And to all the other friends and family who have supported me along the way, you know who you are.

Thank you.

ABOUT THE AUTHOR

Bella has worked in mental health since 2010. She is a registered mental health nurse and integrative psychotherapeutic counsellor. Her previous roles were as a key worker for Mind and Kids Company; a nurse consultant for Save the Children; a family support worker in London prisons and with detainees seeking asylum; an independent mental health advocate (IMHA); and as a mental health and neurodiversity advisor at the University of Oxford.

Bella currently practices as a private therapist, a specialist mental health mentor, and as a mental health advisor and practitioner in the theatre industry.